DYNAMICS
of
FITNESS
and
HEALTH

Sixth Edition

F. Compton Jenkins
Bergen Community College

KENDALL/HUNT PUBLISHING COMPANY
2460 Kerper Boulevard P.O. Box 539 Dubuque, Iowa 52004-0539

Page 75

Figure from PHYSICAL EDUCATION: A PROBLEM SOLVING APPROACH
TO HEALTH AND FITNESS by Perry Johnson, Wynn F. Updyke,
Donald C. Stolberg, and Maryellen Schaefer, copyright © 1966 by Holt,
Rinehart and Winston, Inc., reprinted by permission of the publisher.

Previously titled **EXERCISE: For the Health of It**

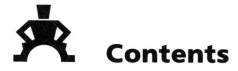

Contents

Acknowledgments

Grateful thanks is extended to the following people who aided in the preparation of this publication:

Mary Pat Boron—an amateur sports photographer whose enthusiasm for both is unbounded.

Thomas Halligan—a student pursuing degree work in exercise science at Bergen Community College and a wrestling enthusiast.

Evette Seidita—a student pursuing degree work in exercise science at Bergen Community College and an exercise instructor.

Robert Thompson—Professor and Program Director, Division of Allied Health & Physical Education at Bergen Community College and one outstanding person.

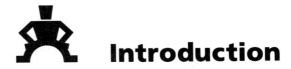 # Introduction

As we approach the 21st century we have become aware that humans continue to radically reshape the environment in which they live. Technological advancements have reduced the effort required to perform daily activities. These changes have contributed greatly to the betterment of society. At the same time, however, major problems have been created, which become evident upon examination of the physical status of the members of society.

There has risen a critical interest in physical activity, which has been an aspect of life minimized by the "machine age." Many pieces of literature have been written that encourage people to participate in various forms of physical activity for a variety of avowed purposes.

This book acquaints readers with information with which they may construct a prudently self-administered exercise program as part of their life-styles. It must be recognized that the needs and interests of people vary. Yet all people share a mutual interest in maintaining their physical selves at an optimal level by using exercise: for the health of it.

The book explores the considerations necessary to develop a fitness level that impacts on health status. To achieve this purpose, chapter material includes information regarding:

▶ The role of exercise in contemporary life-styles

▶ The physical and psychosocial benefits of exercise

▶ Exercise principles and their application

▶ The nature of heart disease and its risk factors

▶ The nature and dangers of obesity

▶ The role of exercise in affecting body weight and heart disease

▶ Considerations regarding diet and calories

▶ The health promotion and disease prevention benefits of exercise

The material presented to the reader represents a condensation of an incredible amount of investigation dealing with exercise. Laboratory experiences are included that help to reinforce concepts presented as well as to provide a better personal understanding of these ideas.

The design and intent of this text is such that an instructor may use the material without being forced into a particular format of presentation. The concepts and laboratory experiences are those believed to be essential to a course of this nature being offered in a situation involving limited facilities, time, and space.

Last, it is hoped that the information presented will help in the classification and consideration of a part of life that is all too often neglected—Exercise: For the Health of It.

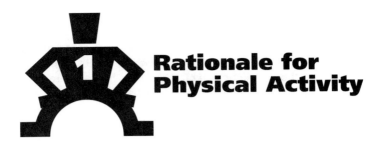

Rationale for Physical Activity

You and Fitness

In the latter half of this century our society has been reacquainted with the meaning and benefit of physical work. We have witnessed the development of an exercise boom. The number of publications, health club memberships, sweat suits, tennis rackets, sport shoes, and bicycles sold all tend to give credence to a curiosity of the American populace regarding exercise. It appears that active Americans—whether dancing, running, swimming, cycling, or pumping iron—are driven by a common goal. They appear to be spurred onward by a belief that exercise transforms their lives in a meaningful and productive fashion. Interestingly, medical, clinical, epidemiological, and anecdotal evidence supports this notion.

Recent survey information indicates that perhaps as many as 83 million Americans are involved in exercise. These surveys support the belief that those who are exercising become more health conscious. Perhaps it is because there may be a distinct relationship between health status and physical fitness. This association may at last be making its impact on a society that cannot afford to sit complacently as the future so rapidly becomes the present.

Most people will acknowledge the need for exercise while at the same time doing little, if anything, to take advantage of what exercise has to offer. It is commonplace to find that most people take better care of, and pay more attention to things they own—cars, wardrobe, stereo systems and the like—than to themselves. For some people the idea of physical fitness equates with a slim waistline and a suntan. One only has to look around to see that most have opted for the suntan.

The human organism needs challenging physical activity. Unfortunately, present day society makes physical effort in life virtually nonexistent. In the past, physical effort was a requisite for life itself. Now, experts fear for the future because our present day society demands much less effort. Technological advancements have created a sedentary, disease-prone society. Degenerative diseases are common today and appear to be directly related to this sedentary existence. This is in keeping with a well-known biological adage that states *"use it or lose it."* Relative to physiological function—the less the

1

body does, the less it can do, and thus it becomes more susceptible to disease and deterioration. The term *hypokinetic disease* is used by Kraus and Raab[1] to describe those afflictions which promote human deterioration through inactivity. The most dramatic example is heart disease, which continues to be the leading cause of death in our society. This is accompanied by other "diseases" that can be profoundly affected by exercise: obesity; low back syndrome; hypertension; diabetes; osteoporosis; and the effects of emotional stress, such as depression.

Ever-mounting evidence suggests that exercise and its corollary, physical fitness, can significantly enhance health status and well-being. Whether fitness can *guarantee* better health remains to be seen. Exercise can provide the basis of a "fitness for life" that may carry with it a greater health status. People are born with a 70-year warranty—*not* a guarantee. Exercise can aid in living a healthier, more abundant, more productive life.

"EXERCISE IS MEDICINE"—according to a survey of 1,750 primary care physicians conducted by the journal *The Physician and Sportsmedicine*. They prescribe exercise for weight control (95%), cardiac rehabilitation (94%), depression (85%), low back pain (83%), arthritis (80%), diabetes (80%), anxiety (60%), chronic obstructive pulmonary disease (58%), asthma (56%), and chemical dependence (43%).

The most frequently prescribed modes (types) of exercise are walking (97%), swimming (82%), bicycling (67%), strength training (67%), and running (46%).

One important consideration to bear in mind is that exercise need not mean engaging in competitive ventures like athletics. A distinct difference exists between what is now understood as *sports fitness* as opposed to *health-related fitness.*

Individuals tend to relate exercise with competitive sports like football, baseball, tennis, and others while disregarding the basic tenet that not all exercise is the same. Competitive athletics encompasses many requisites that are specific to a particular sport, that is, sports fitness. Any exercise undertaken with a competitive orientation necessitates high levels of skill, preparation, motivation, and related physical attributes. The qualities that create and sustain high athletic performance are largely genetically determined.

Favorite sports may require high levels of skill, superb judgment, or steel-like nerves but may make little contribution to fitness. If whatever you do in the form of "exercise" makes no strenuous demands on your body, requires little prolonged exertion or in no other way helps to improve your heart, lungs, and muscular system, your exercise is not contributing to health-related fitness—fitness for life.

Unless you anticipate turning "pro" or becoming a member of an Olympic team, you should seek to develop overall fitness, not just timing, swing, or speed. There is a distinct difference between specific sport training and exercising for fitness and health. It is not unusual to find a pro athlete who is below average in health-related fitness but second to none in his or her sport specialty skills.

The goal for most people should not be athletic excellence (that may never be achieved) but, rather, physical conditioning for the demands of daily life.

With each passing year your basic physical condition—fitness—becomes increasingly important. No one ever died from skinny legs or underdeveloped biceps, but thousands become victims of heart disease, the consequences of obesity, the ravages of stress, and generally poor physical condition.

Total fitness should be your most important consideration, and it can only be achieved when the body is strong and viable. It incorporates a balance of living that integrates mental, physical, and emotional optimums. Exercise is not a panacea for each individual's needs, but it does make an indispensable contribution. Very simply, exercise can make you look better, feel better, and function better.

> "If all you do is sit and read,
> all you get is smart and soft."
>
> —Scott Carpenter, NASA Astronaut

The following will serve to indicate the impact that exercise may have on the health and fitness of each individual. It is a summary of evidence concerning the relationships of exercise and health from *Exercise and Health: A Point of View.*[2]

1. **Studies Concerning the General Values of Exercise Indicate:**

   a. That regular physical activity produces organic changes, particularly in the lungs and circulatory system, some of which improve function for normal living and protect against stress and strain.
   b. That systematic muscular exercise leads to the increase of height, shoulder breadth, and strength, beyond changes resulting from maturation.
   c. That in young adulthood systematic exercise increases body weight and vital capacity of growing youths.
   d. That regular physical activity will eventually increase the density of the bones of the body and increase their resistance to stress and strain.
   e. That with regular training muscles increase in size, strength, and capacity for work, thus making the accomplishment of regular daily activities easier.

2. **Studies Relating to the Effect of Exercise on Aging Indicate:**

   a. That despite the popular belief to the contrary, the life expectancy of an athlete (person exposed to vigorous exercise) is as high as the average life expectancy and, excluding accidents, is probably higher than the average.

   b. That the percentage of athletes that are afflicted with degenerative disease is probably lower than for the general population.

   c. That there is good reason to believe that proper physical activity can significantly delay the aging process.

   d. That regular proper exercise can help to preserve physical and mental capacities longer than otherwise.

3. **Studies Relating to the Heart and Exercise Indicate:**

   a. That vigorous exercise reasonably applied under rational conditions will not damage healthy young hearts.

   b. That proper exercise as a way of life helps to keep healthy hearts healthy and to prevent the onset of cardiovascular disease.

   c. That proper exercise as a way of life may help to lessen the severity of and make recovery from cardiovascular disease more likely.

   d. That medically prescribed exercise after an appropriate period following a heart attack can frequently hasten recovery and rehabilitation.

4. **Studies Concerning Exercise in Rehabilitation Indicate:**

   a. That proper medical application of early ambulation and physical activity in convalescence can reduce hospital readmissions and shorten the recovery period by substantial amounts.

   b. That properly prescribed and administered exercise, as one phase of treatment, can help muscle tone, strength, and endurance and prevent certain complications.

   c. That in certain conditions, properly prescribed exercises can help in the development of compensatory functions and adaptations (such as the regeneration of nerves or the building of an alternate blood supply).

Exercise: A Matter of Choice

The decisions to be made in life are limitless and by no means easy. Decisions must often be made today that may not show their true impact for weeks, months, or even years to come. Making a choice regarding the inclusion of exercise in one's life is such a decision. The quality and quantity of life ahead very much depends on habits that are begun in the present: *If you could omit heredity, the two factors that would influence your well-being the most are exercise and diet.*

Lack of exercise and resulting low levels of fitness are very important risk factors in disease and early death. Large volumes of exercise are not necessary to produce significant improvement in health status; in fact, moderate exercise and fitness levels seem to offer considerable health benefit. Thirty-five to 70 million U.S. adults may be at risk because of low activity and fitness. This constitutes a public health problem of major proportions.

Including exercise as a life-style habit can make a substantial impact on both immediate and lifelong health status. The choice and commitment is up to each individual.

Summary

The human body has a physiological need for exercise, which serves to enhance functional capacity to optimal levels. This, in turn, can affect one's health status and the tendency to resist the effects of degenerative diseases so prevalent in our sedentary society. This list of benefits that can be derived from exercise and resulting increased fitness seem to transcend the physical and begin to enhance mental and emotional factors as well.

Research supports several significant conclusions:

▶ Low levels of exercise and fitness are important risk factors for disease and early death.

▶ Relatively low levels of exercise produce definitive benefit: A little exercise is better than no exercise.

▶ The basic beliefs about exercise and its benefit rest on solid scientific foundation.

Exercise: A Health Habit

Scientific study of the responses of the body to exercise began early in this century and has expanded since the 1950s. When the results of these studies are examined, there is strong evidence that regular exercise is an important health habit. Generally, it is revealed that sedentary lifestyles and low levels of physical fitness are associated with higher rates of morbidity and mortality. Recently, a study directed by Dr. Steven Blair at the Institute for Aerobics Research involving 10,224 men and 3,120 women covering a period of eight years was completed. In this study fitness was assessed via a treadmill stress test and participants were grouped in fitness categories based on results: low fitness level (bottom 20%); moderate fitness level (middle 40%); and high fitness level (upper 40%). When the data was analyzed, it was determined that men and women in the low fitness category were more than twice as likely to die from cancer, cardiovascular disease, and from all causes combined than those in the moderate fitness group. The lowest death rates from all causes were found in the high fitness group. When factors such as cigarette smoking, high cholesterol, family history of heart disease, high blood sugar levels, and high body mass index (overweight and obesity) were statistically adjusted for cause of death, it was found that low fitness level is just as important as other risk factors in early mortality; that is, low physical fitness is an independent risk factor for early death.

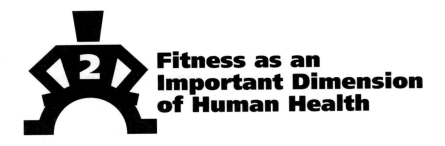

Fitness as an Important Dimension of Human Health

What Is Physical Fitness?

Physical fitness is a term often used but little understood by many people, because fitness is very difficult to define. A widely accepted concept of fitness involves a condition of living that characterizes the degree to which a person is able to function efficiently in daily life. Doctors may indicate that fitness could substitute for health; athletes may indicate that fitness is synonymous with skill, speed, and power; models, like Christie Brinkley, may indicate that fitness requires a slim, shapely figure. In essence, each is correct by describing one part of what fitness includes. It must be remembered that fitness does not come in a "have" or "have not" package. Everyone possesses those qualities described by the doctor, athlete, and model. Those qualities and many others all describe fitness as a quality of life, with only the amount or degree showing variation from person to person. As described previously, some parts of fitness directly affect health status whereas others primarily affect performance or skill-related fitness (sports/athletics).

Each person should possess those qualities of fitness which support "health." These *health-related fitness qualities* are:

▶ **Cardiorespiratory Efficiency**—The optimal functional capacity of the heart, lungs, and blood vessels.

▶ **Body Weight—Body Composition Measures**—Optimal total body weight and lean/fat proportions.

▶ **Musculoskeletal Efficiency** (strength, endurance, and flexibility)— Optimal levels of muscular function accompanied by optimal ranges of motion and integrity of body segments.

7

Skill-related fitness includes qualities that support a variety of movements necessary to perform all sports efficiently but are not necessarily related to one's medical or health status. These elements create **neuromuscular coordination,** commonly called skill. The components that enable skilled movement include:

Balance: The ability to maintain neuromuscular control of the body position. Balance is important to most neuromuscular tasks but is critical in activities such as gymnastics, springboard diving, and activities in which an opponent attempts to upset you, such as in football or hockey.

Power: The ability to transfer energy into force at a fast rate of speed (explosive body movement). Power is needed in such activities as sprinting or hitting a baseball or tennis ball and can be developed by placing a resistance against the muscle group (such as weighted shoes for sprinters) or by developing muscles in the wrist or forearm when hitting an object.

Speed: The ability to move the entire body or body part rapidly. Speed is important in many motor activities such as basketball, baseball, track, and soccer. The improvement of speed depends on improved running techniques and the greater strength and endurance development of the specific muscles used in the activity. Improvement is limited to the anatomical differences of the person, which is dictated by overall body build. Big-boned people with large girth through the middle of the body would have a speed disadvantage.

Agility: The ability to change the direction or the position of the body rapidly. Agility depends on elements of speed and power. Most activities that involve a response to a stimulus such as a ball hit or served to either side of you would require the power to push off and change direction and the speed necessary to pursue the object. Agility can be improved by requiring the body to change direction in a repetitive manner.

Reaction Time: The time elapsing between a stimulus and the body's reaction to the stimulus. Reaction time would be important to a sprinter as he or she responds to the gun or an outfielder who responds to the crack of the bat. Constant repetition of the stimulus can help to improve the reaction time.

Kinesthetic Sense: The ability of the individual to perceive the relationship of his or her body to the ground and space and make proper adjustments. Kinesthetic sense would be particularly important to a diver or gymnast who must land at a particular point on the ground or in the pool. Constant repetition and refinement can develop this aspect of skill.

Skill is the ability to perform a task with ease and efficiency. The aspects of motor activity can be improved through repetition that emphasizes correct movement patterns. Practice will improve performance only if the reinforcement is a correct one.

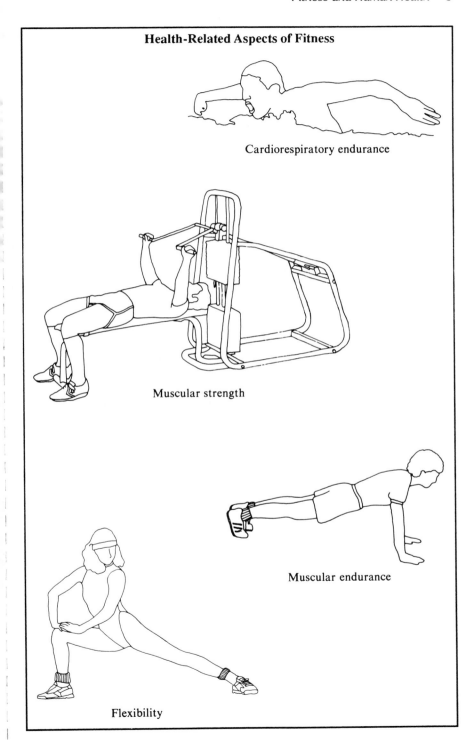

Health-Related Aspects of Fitness

Cardiorespiratory endurance

Muscular strength

Muscular endurance

Flexibility

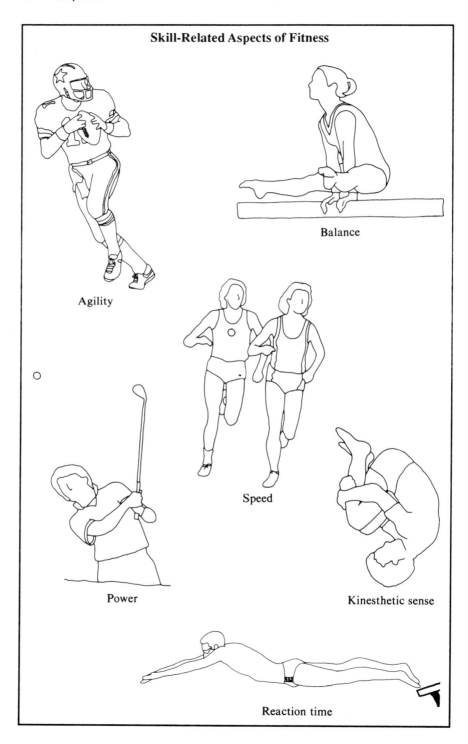

Skill-Related Aspects of Fitness

Agility

Balance

Speed

Power

Kinesthetic sense

Reaction time

Neuromuscular coordination can contribute to the other aspects of fitness by providing a satisfying motor activity that could develop strength, endurance, and flexibility as well as provide a pleasant daily experience.

Since only a few of the components of fitness have direct bearing on health status, they become the focus in the pursuit of optimal physical fitness. This is the most favorable health which is needed for the enthusiastic undertaking of daily responsibilities and tasks as well as recreational and exercise activities. It is optimal physical fitness that aids in creating a life-style experience that the unfit cannot enjoy or understand. People who possess optimal physical fitness tend to *look better, feel better, and experience good health, which all contribute to the quality of life.*

Optimal cardiorespiratory function, musculoskeletal efficiency, and body composition are the most important components of fitness for health.

Strength is probably the most familiar component of fitness. It is defined as the maximum amount of force that can be produced by muscle. Strength is important to all sports and daily activities. Whether one is exercising or carrying groceries, muscular strength supports the activity. Strength training (weight training) results in some enlargement (hypertrophy) of muscle and a resulting increase in the ability to produce force.

Muscular endurance is the ability of muscle to produce repetitive movement over extended periods of time. The ability to do sit-ups, push-ups, shovel snow, wash windows, and paint are all examples of when muscular endurance becomes very important.

Flexibility is the ability to move the joints of the body. Bending, stretching, twisting all involve the use of muscle to move a skeletal joint throughout a range of motion. Maintenance of flexibility at optimal levels is important so that the susceptibility to injury may be reduced.

Body composition is the component of fitness that relates to total body weight and its parts—fat and lean body weight. The amounts of fat and lean tissue, like muscle and bone, form a proportion that is more important than total body weight. The relative amounts of lean body weight and fat weight are very much related to health and fitness.

Cardiorespiratory efficiency is the most important fitness component. The ability of the body to supply and deliver oxygen is the key to life. All activities depend on muscle function, which in turn is determined by adequate oxygen supply. Efficient functioning of the heart and lungs is a basic requirement for the enjoyment of activities that support fitness, as well as health.

The Effects of Exercise

There is no shortcut to fitness. We *must* exercise. Regular exercise has been found to produce many beneficial effects.

The effects of exercise can be transitory (short term) and have little long-term consequence or can be long-lasting with many significant lifetime benefits. Let's examine the differences of some easily observed changes.

Immediate Effects: Changes in the body that occur during or immediately after physical activity. The nature of the change will depend on the intensity of the activity.

▶ Increased pulse rate: The heart will usually beat faster during all physical activity. The increase will be minimal if the activity does not call for significant exertion and could be as high as twice the resting pulse rate if the activity calls for near maximum effort. This increased rate enables the heart to pump more blood, containing oxygen, to the cells during the period of need.

▶ Increased consumption of oxygen: The body cells will quickly exhaust the available oxygen and will require more oxygen to enable a continuation of the activity.

▶ Increased respiration rate: The lungs will increase their activity as breathing becomes more rapid to supply the oxygen needed by the body for a particular activity.

▶ Dilation of blood vessels in skin: The smaller blood vessels of the skin become dilated (enlarged) to aid in cooling the body. This may cause the skin to take on a flushed or red color, especially noticeable in the face.

▶ Perspiration: A higher body core temperature occurs during exercise and perspiration enables the body to eliminate excessive heat through evaporation. This phenomenon is basic in the mechanism of heat loss from the body.

The immediate effects of exercise are quickly dispelled during a rest period. Indeed, we all experience the immediate effects of exercise regardless of fitness level.

Long-Term (Training) Effects: Changes that occur in the body after regular exercise. The time span will vary but usually consists of exercise programs done regularly (3–5 times per week) for a period of several weeks. The beneficial changes will depend on the specificity of the exercise program in determining the training effect. These changes include:

▶ Increased size of the heart: The heart, as any muscle, will increase in overall size in response to exercise. The walls will become thicker and stronger allowing for greater efficiency and increased work capacity.

▶ Increased stroke volume: All chambers of the heart will become capable of pumping increased amounts of blood each time they contract. This amount of blood pumped with each contraction of the heart is called the stroke volume. The heart muscle can get more blood to the body with each beat as the left ventricle forces more blood out of the heart with each contraction (called a systole).

▶ Decreased resting pulse rate: The body's need for blood will be satisfied by fewer beats per minute as each beat represents greater stroke volume. The heart is capable of supplying enough blood by performing less work. This increased efficiency can be noticed by a decrease in the number of beats per minute.

▶ Decreased exercise pulse rate: The maximum heart rate will decrease with age, but conditioned people will have lower exercise pulse rates regardless of age. The efficiency of the heart is reflected during exercise by having to beat at a lower rate.

▶ Faster pulse rate recovery: The exercised person will have a faster return to normal pulse rate after an exercise bout. The increased pulse rate recovery occurs because you are capable of providing the cells with more oxygenated blood and removing fatigue products after exercise. The cell needs will be satisfied more quickly than in the deconditioned individual.

▶ Faster oxygen debt recovery: The respiratory system is capable of an increased ability to exchange air with an increased ability to absorb oxygen from the air. The body will be provided with enough oxygen for the need to be satisfied.

▶ Increased ability to sustain activity for long periods of time: An increase in the length of exercise time will be readily apparent due to increased physiological efficiency in the production of energy, supply of oxygen, and removal of fatigue products.

▶ A decrease in the amount of body fat: Exercise that uses entire body movement will place significantly greater demands on physical work capacity. Consequently the body must supply more energy, which is achieved through various metabolic processes. A strenuous exercise program could burn off as much as 10 times the calories needed at rest. Exercise, in conjunction with proper diet, would aid in reducing body fat because the additional energy would be supplied from stored fat.

▶ Increased size of muscle fibers: The muscle fibers will increase in size, providing greater tone and muscle definition. The amount of increase will depend on the intensity of the exercise and will be subject to the anatomical differences between individuals and between the sexes.

▶ Increased muscular strength: Exercise programs that place increasing stress on the musculature will produce impressive strength gains in the muscle or muscle groups being exercised. Skeletal bone density will also increase, therefore helping to prevent osteoporosis.

▶ Increased muscular endurance: Exercise programs that increase the number of repetitions a muscle or muscle group performs will produce an increased capacity of the muscles to continue in the particular exercise before muscle fatigue occurs.

▶ Reduced emotional stress: Regular, continuous exercise provides an outlet for stress and enables you to have a satisfying psychological experience while gaining physical benefit as well.

When one considers the impact of activity on health it is easy to see that exercise is where prevention and rehabilitation cross over. The following list of factors that affect health are also affected by exercise—for prevention or rehabilitation:

▶ lower blood pressure

▶ cessation of smoking

▶ lower cholesterol

▶ complete body conditioning

▶ diabetes

▶ stress management

▶ control of body weight and fatness

▶ control of the effects of mental/emotional stress

"There is more to health than just feeling good—GET FIT"

David E. Jenkins, Physical Education Teacher
Ridgewood Public Schools, New Jersey

A Summary of the Adaptation Effects of Endurance Training after Several Weeks

Measure	Change
Myocardial size and weight	Increase
Muscle capillarization	Increase
Percentage of body fat	Decrease
Hemoglobin (carries oxygen)	Increase
Vital Capacity (lung capacity)	Increase
Serum Cholesterol	No change/or decrease
HDL Cholesterol	Increase
LDL Cholesterol	Decrease
Triglycerides	Decrease
Total Blood Volume	Increase
Systolic Blood Pressure	Decrease/no change
Diastolic Blood Pressure	Decrease/no change
Heart rate (Resting)	Decrease
Stroke volume	Increase

Why Do People Exercise?

Why then, is fitness, the result of exercise, important? Surveys would produce a listing of hundreds of reasons. Basically, there are only two:

1. **To Create a Physical Change**—to lose weight/fat; to reduce blood pressure; to reduce the effects of stress; to reduce a diabetic condition; to reduce osteoporosis; to reduce cholesterol; to increase strength; to increase endurance; to reduce the effects of smoking; to decrease fatigue; to reduce low back pain; and to feel better.

2. **To Prevent a Physical Change**—to prevent weight gain/fat gain; to prevent increases in blood pressure; to prevent the deterioration related to stress; to prevent adult diabetes; to prevent osteoporosis; to prevent increases in cholesterol; to prevent losses of strength/endurance; to prevent low back pain; and to prevent feeling lousy.

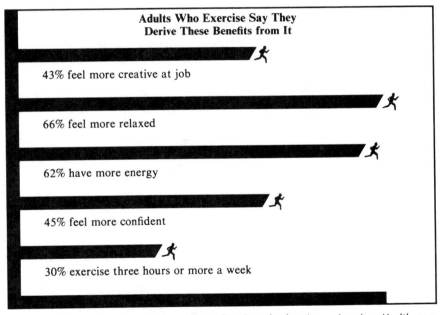

Adults Who Exercise Say They Derive These Benefits from It

43% feel more creative at job

66% feel more relaxed

62% have more energy

45% feel more confident

30% exercise three hours or more a week

These statistics are based on findings by a Gallup Organization, Inc.—*American Health* magazine poll of 1,019 Americans in November, 1984. Reprinted with permission from AMERICAN HEALTH: FITNESS OF BODY AND MIND, copyright 1986, *American Health Partners Inc.*

Summary

Physical fitness characterizes the degree to which a person is able to function efficiently. Each person has different fitness needs depending on his or her individual life-style. The components usually needed for good fitness are muscular strength, muscular endurance, flexibility, cardiovascular endurance, and neuromuscular coordination. Neuromuscular coordination is synonymous with motor (athletic) ability and includes the elements of balance, power, speed, agility, reaction time, and kinesthetic sense.

Exercise produces immediate effects to the body such as perspiration, elevated pulse rate, and flushed face. These effects disappear during a resting phase. The long-term effects of exercise programs done at least three times a week for several weeks include an increase in heart size, increased stroke volume, decreased resting pulse rate, faster recovery rate of the heart, increased ability to sustain the heart for long periods of time, increased caloric burn off, increased muscle tone, increased muscle strength, and increased muscle endurance.

Most of us have learned some commonsense "health rules" from our parents, grandparents, aunts, uncles, and teachers, ranging from "smoking is bad for you" and "breakfast is the most important meal of the day" to "don't get fat." Research from all areas of the medical and physiological areas implicates many health habits as factors in creating a wide range of major disease problems. One such health habit is exercise/physical activity.

When consideration is made relative to the result of exercise/physical activity, fitness, it is reasonable to expect improved health and longevity. An editorial in the Journal of the American Medical Association in 1978 supported the concept that the most promising factor for improving public health rests with what people can be motivated to do for themselves.

Fitness: Interest and Action

Eighty percent of American adults say that they are either "somewhat satisfied" or "very satisfied" with their physical condition, according to a recent survey completed by the University of Michigan, Ann Arbor. The director of the study, Dr. Christine L. Brooks, finds these responses alarming because the vast majority of these individuals never did any form of physical activity that would even begin to challenge their cardiovascular systems. The most frequent activity indicated was walking. This study was supported by findings reported by the National Center for Health Statistics Survey of 1979 which indicated that 58 percent of adults do not exercise regularly, but 80 percent consider themselves to be as active or more active than others of the same age group.

Additionally, relative to understanding exercise, most Americans are not knowledgeable about the scientific recommendations for frequency, intensity, and duration of exercise. The University of Michigan study raises significant questions about the popularity of exercise; the participation rate by adults; and the scientific understanding of exercise.

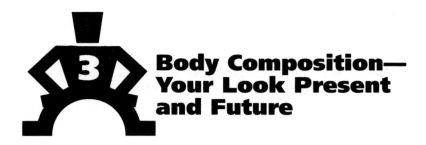

Body Composition—Your Look Present and Future

In addition to being of major importance to physiological efficiency, psychological well-being, and self-image, weight control is probably the most abused aspect of self-maintenance. This is due to basic misunderstanding about the causes of physical change, which is why obesity continues to be a major medical and personal fitness problem.

Diet fads, gimmicks, and quackery gross more than $100 million each year. The public has indicated its gullibility by spending some $500 million each year on short-term cure-all gadgets for fitness and fat control.

Since obesity ranks as such a major problem—mentally, emotionally, and physically—some consideration should be given to what causes the onset of this condition. Obesity probably has no one single cause but rather is caused by an interplay of a number of factors. From this standpoint it may be said that there are various causes in various people, but these factors acting alone or in any combination have one final manifestation—increased fat storage leading toward obesity.

Presently, four principal factors appear to control weight gain and potential obesity. When considered as an *obesity syndrome,* these factors work together to produce one inevitable result: increased fatness. These factors are:

▶ Genetic influences—those inherited tendencies toward obesity which include physical and biochemical markers, that is, where fat tends to be stored (a genetic fat pattern) and lipoprotein lipase (LPL), an enzyme that enhances fat storage.

▶ Sedentary life-style—inactivity that starts early in the childhood years and has lifelong consequences affecting caloric expenditure and body composition.

▶ Overeating—insensitivity to the energy equation, which involves calories consumed relative to calories expended.

▶ Psychological inducements—those associations made with food, that is, love, security, comfort, socializing, and the use of food as a stress escape mechanism.

Physical Appearance

We are all products of **heredity** and **environment.** These two factors in life have determined everything that we have been, what we are now, and will determine what we will be; in other words, what we get from parents and what we do with what we get.

Since the problem of weight control seems to focus on physical appearance, it is important to understand why you appear as you do.

Somatotyping

Your physical appearance is called a **somatotype** (body build). There are three classifications of somatotypes—**endomorph, mesomorph,** and **ectomorph.** Each has specific characteristics based on the relative predominance of bone, fat, and muscle. Some of the general characteristics that apply more commonly to these body builds are:

Endomorph—A large soft bulging body, a "pear-shaped" appearance, short arms and legs, most of the body weight centered around the hips and abdomen, lack of bony angularity, and heavy fat pad distribution. The endomorph's response to conditioning is slow, but great improvements are possible. See page 24 for detailed characteristics.

Mesomorph—Solid, muscular, large-boned physique, most of the body weight is away from the abdominal area, wide shoulders, narrow hips, and well-muscled throughout. Mesomorphs respond very well to conditioning. See page 25 for detailed characteristics.

Ectomorph—Slender bodies and a slight build, very little body fat, light musculature, long arms and legs, bony in appearance, narrow chest and hips, and generally linear in appearance. Ectomorphs' response to conditioning may be slow with greater success in endurance activities and those involving support of the body weight and little body contact. See page 26 for detailed characteristics.

Assessing Body Build

It should be obvious that most people have some characteristics of each body type because everyone has certain amounts of bone, fat, and muscle. Dr. William Sheldon, M.D., developed the most comprehensive system of somatotyping, that is, classifying physical appearances. His system is based on the use of a number scale (1–7) indicating to what degree characteristics from each category are present in an individual's appearance. Using the scale, the number 1 would indicate the lowest degree and the number 7 would indicate the highest degree of represented characteristics. Therefore, a somatotype is represented by three numbers: The first always indicates endomorphy, the middle number always indicates mesomorphy, and the third number always indicates ectomorphy. For example, if you were to give a somatotype to Santa Claus, the first number may be 7—indicating maximum "roundness"; the middle number may be 3—indicating "muscularity"; and the third number may be 1—indicating "linearity." So the somatotype becomes 7–3–1, a numerical picture of a physical appearance. The body type named depends on where the highest number is found. Santa Claus would be called an endomorph, since the highest number is in the first category.

This body type classification system is subjectively determined and will vary with expertise in the area. The prime concern is to recognize readily apparent individual characteristics and to use them in personalizing an exercise program. Your somatotype and its change is one of many factors that aid in the development of a realistic self-image.

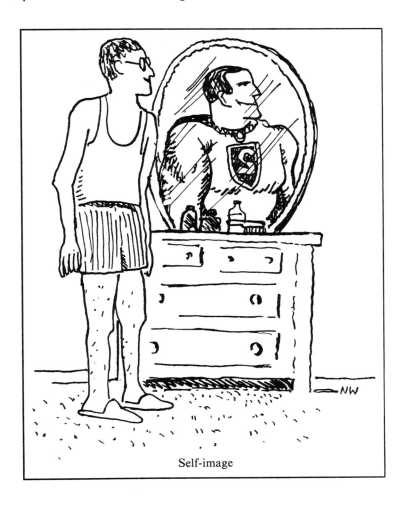

Self-image

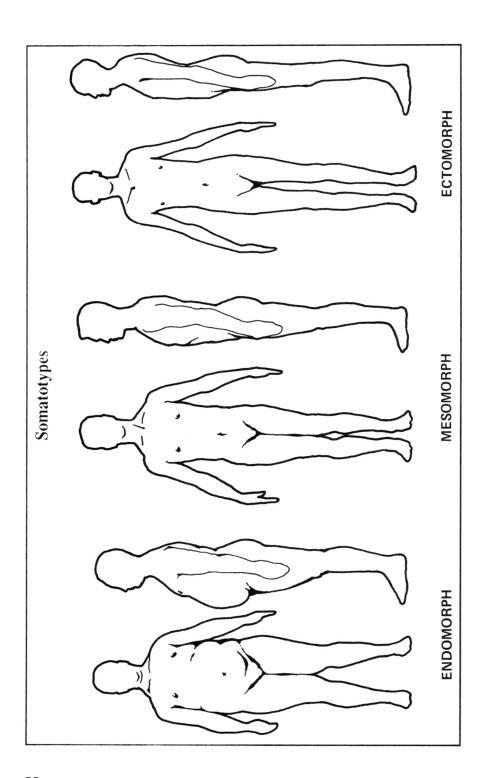

Somatotypes

ECTOMORPH

MESOMORPH

ENDOMORPH

22

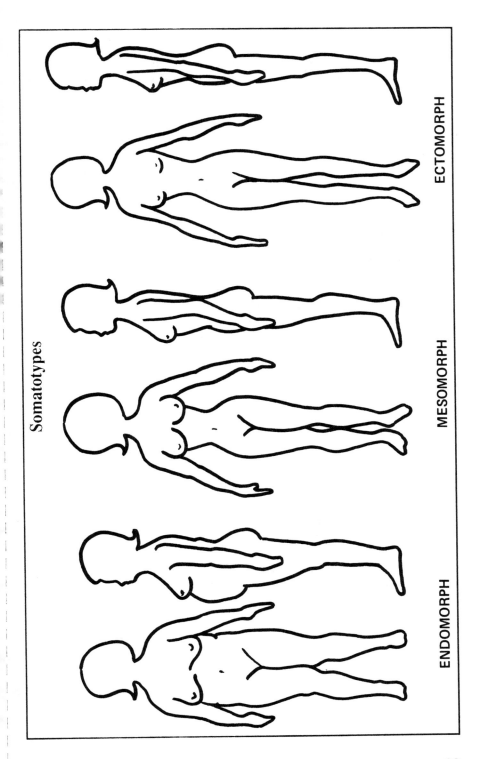

Somatotypes

ECTOMORPH

MESOMORPH

ENDOMORPH

The fitness/health needs and problems of each type vary. Endomorphic individuals encounter an ever-present weight control problem and require special efforts in this direction. Mesomorphic individuals are prone to increases in body weight, usually reflecting additional fatness particularly when age increases and activity level drops sharply. Ectomorphic individuals seem to have less to worry about regarding body weight but may experience problems that are largely strength related.

No one is immune to weight gain—especially when the gain involves an increase in the amount of body fat (adipose).

Lateral Body Type (Endomorphic) Morphological Characteristics

I. General Appearance
- Large, soft, bulging body
- Thick body segments, anteroposteriorly
- Mass concentrated toward center
- Roundness and softness of body
- Anteroposterior and lateral diameters tend toward equality in the head, neck, trunk, and limbs
- Hair is fine and sparse

II. Segments
1. Head, Neck, Face
   - Large, round head
   - Short, thick neck
   - Neck forms obtuse angle with chin in lateral plane
   - Wide, round face; wide, low palate

2. Thoracic Trunk
   - Broad, thick chest
   - Wide costal angle
   - Some fatty breasts
   - Relatively straight spine
   - Postural defects of shoulders not common
   - Clavicular and scapulae hollows well padded

3. Arms, Shoulders, Hands
   - Short arms, relatively
   - Short forearms, relatively
   - Limbs taper from "hammy" upperarms to small hands and wrists

Reprinted by permission of the American Alliance for Health, Physical Education, Recreation and Dance, 1900 Association Drive, Reston, Va 22091. Division of Girls and Women's Sports Research Reports, "Women in Sports," 1973.

▶ High, square shoulders
▶ Smooth feminine musculature with no sharp muscle contours, viz.: deltoids and trapezeii
▶ Short fingers, relatively

4. Abdominal Trunk and Pelvis
    ▶ Large abdomen, full above navel and pendulous
    ▶ Long abdomen from sternum to pubis
    ▶ Thick A-P depth at navel
    ▶ Relatively straight lumbar spine

5. Legs, Feet, Buttocks
    ▶ Short legs, relatively
    ▶ Heavy, fat buttocks with no dimpling or muscle outlines
    ▶ Short forelegs, relatively
    ▶ Heavy, "hammy" thighs
    ▶ Large, smooth calves
    ▶ Feet small and weakness common
    ▶ Foot defects common

Heavy Athletic Body Type (Mesomorphic) Morphological Characteristics

I. General Appearance
    ▶ A squareness and hardness of body
    ▶ Rugged, prominent, massive muscles
    ▶ Large, prominent bones
    ▶ Transverse diameters of shoulders, forearms, and calves are large, but A-P diameters are less than in endomorphic types
    ▶ Central concentration of mass is absent
    ▶ Long and upright trunk, proportions variable
    ▶ Skin is thick and coarse with conspicuous pores; holds good tan, small wrinkles infrequent
    ▶ Hair is coarse, thick, or sparse

II. Segments

    1. Head, Neck, Face
        ▶ Head variable in size and shape but often cubicle with thick and dense bones
        ▶ Facial bones are prominent, viz.: cheekbones, supraorbital ridges; square jaws

Reprinted by permission of the American Alliance for Health, Physical Education, Recreation and Dance, 1900 Association Drive, Reston, Va 22091. Division of Girls and Women's Sports Research Reports, "Women in Sports," 1973.

- ► Facial mass great compared to cephalic mass
- ► Fairly long, strong neck with great transverse diameter compared to anteroposterior diameter
- ► Hair on head variable

2. Thoracic Trunk
   - ► Predominates in volume over abdominal volume
   - ► Wide thorax at apex
   - ► Little thoracic curve in spine
   - ► Ribs—strong and heavy

3. Arms, Shoulders, Hands
   - ► Shoulders seem low with trapezium and deltoidius muscles prominent
   - ► Broad shoulders
   - ► Clavicles heavy and prominent
   - ► Muscular upperarm, no "hamming"
   - ► Massive forearms, wrists, hands, and fingers
   - ► Upperarm and forearm evenly proportioned

4. Abdominal Trunk and Pelvis
   - ► Abdomen is large and heavily muscled ripples show
   - ► Slender, low waist
   - ► Pelvis sturdy and powerful with broad hips

Linear Body Type (Ectomorphic) Morphological Characteristics

I. General Appearance
   - ► Thin body segments, anteroposteriorly
   - ► Decentralization of structure
   - ► Linearity, thinness
   - ► Frail, delicate body structure
   - ► Small, thin-diameter bones
   - ► Undernourished appearance
   - ► Small trunk, long limbs
   - ► Profuse hair, baldness uncommon

II. Segments
   1. Head, Neck, Face
      - ► Relatively large cranium
      - ► Bulbous forehead
      - ► Small face, pointed chin, sharp nose

Reprinted by permission of the American Alliance for Health, Physical Education, Recreation and Dance, 1900 Association Drive, Reston, Va 22091. Division of Girls and Women's Sports Research Reports, "Women in Sports," 1973.

▶ Long, slender neck
▶ Poke neck common
▶ Lips delicate, thin, dry, pale
▶ Abundant hair on head

2. Thoracic Trunk
   ▶ Narrow thorax, long compared to abdomen
   ▶ Acute costal angle
   ▶ Thin chest depth
   ▶ Clavicular hollows marked, clavicles prominent
   ▶ Winged scapulae, forward shoulders marked
   ▶ Ribs prominent
   ▶ Kyphosis, marked S-curve

3. Arms, Shoulders, Hands
   ▶ Long arms, relatively
   ▶ Long forearms, compared to upperarm
   ▶ Thin upperarms, muscles not marked
   ▶ Shoulder droop and round shoulders marked
   ▶ Thin forearms
   ▶ Long thin hands
   ▶ Inconspicuous knuckles

4. Abdominal Trunk and Pelvis
   ▶ Flat abdomen, hollow above navel
   ▶ Short abdomen, protrusion common below navel
   ▶ Thin anteroposterior depth at navel
   ▶ Lordosis, marked S-curve

5. Legs, Feet, Buttocks
   ▶ Long legs, relatively
   ▶ Inconspicuous buttocks
   ▶ Long forelegs, relatively
   ▶ Thin thighs, muscles not marked
   ▶ Calves relatively thin
   ▶ Feet thin and long

Body Weight and Body Composition

Your **total body weight (TBW)** will generally be related to your somatotype due to the predominance of fat, muscle, or bone. If you are like most Americans your weight will receive considerable attention during your lifetime, and well it should. Most people rely on a bathroom scale and a height-weight chart to determine if they are underweight, proper weight, or overweight. Although this method is easy and certainly accessible, it may also be very misleading.

Overweight and Overfat

When using a scale and height-weight charts you are finding only total body weight (TBW), not how much of that weight is bone, fat, and muscle. This becomes important because the so-called ideal weight on a chart may vary as much as twenty pounds. The important consideration is not only body weight but also how much of the total is lean body weight and how much of the total is fat (adipose). **Lean body weight (LBW)** is composed of essentially four elements: bone, muscle, viscera (internal organs), and fluids. The other component of total weight is **fat weight (FW),** called adipose tissue.

When using height-weight charts a general guideline for determining overweight is to follow a "10% rule." If you exceed a recommended weight by more than 10% you are considered to be **overweight.** However, it does not reveal whether this "excess weight" is due predominantly to lean body weight or too much fat.

A "20% rule" exists as well in relation to body weight and weight charts. If you exceed a recommended weight by more than 20%, you are considered to be **obese.**

Although the terms overweight and overfat (obese) are used interchangeably, they are not necessarily synonymous. Overweight reflects only total body weight, not what composes that total. Overfat reflects an aspect of body composition that represents the presence of too much adipose as part of the total.

Many individuals may be overweight but not overfat. Some individuals, like professional football players, for example, may be 20 to 30 lb or more above a recommended weight (height-weight table). Technically they are overweight, but most of that weight is lean body weight with just a small percentage of fat. Consequently, these individuals would not be classified as overfat.

Determining How Much Fat and Lean

How does one determine the composition of their total body weight, that is, how much lean weight and how much fat weight? There are a number of methods, which vary in sophistication. Probably, the most simple method is to stand in front of a mirror with minimal or no clothes on. Mirrors tend to tell the truth.

Other relatively common methods include the following:

1. **Hydrostatic Weighing**—a comparison of your weight while you are under water to your scale weight. This is considered the best method but it is not very practical.

2. **Skinfold Measurement**—a caliper is used to measure the thickness of skin and subcutaneous (under skin) fat. The thickness is measured at various points on the body and results yields an estimate of total fat. This method is very practical and is considered good because most of your fat is subcutaneous, about 60%.

3. **Ultrasound, Light Wave, and Electrical Impedance**—all are results of "high-tech" advancements and involve sophisticated equipment. The amount of fat is determined by the speed of sound, light, or electricity through fat and muscle, which have different densities.

4. **Body Mass Index and Ponderal Index**—are mathematical methods based on height and weight. These are very easy to do but do not allow for differences in somatotype.

How Much Body Fat?

As indicated in a previous section, a certain amount of body fat is always present in each individual. Body fat is classified as either essential fat or storage fat. The **essential fat** is that located in various organs of the body such as the heart, lungs, liver, spleen, kidneys, intestines, and brain. **Storage fat** accumulates in adipose tissue found surrounding internal organs and subcutaneously. A certain amount of fat is both necessary and valuable to adequate physiological function. However, a point does exist at which an individual can possess too much fat. These guidelines are generally followed: Mature men have an average of 15% to 20% body fat, whereas mature women have an average of 25% body fat. The relative standards for both sexes reflecting overfatness would be above 20% for men and above 30% for women. The disparity between the two standards for obesity exists due to a greater amount of essential fat that is found in the female. Dr. Kenneth M. Cooper, author of *Aerobics* and *The New Aerobics,* recommends the following percentages of body fat as maximum for men and women, respectively, 18% and 22%. A high percentage of body fat may occur at any total body weight and has a significant effect on normal physiological function-health. (To determine body composition, body weight, and body fat levels, see laboratory 3 in the back section of the text.)

It must be remembered that although guidelines exist for both weight and fatness, *adjustments must be made on an individual basis* that reflects body build or somatotype. For example, a person who is an endomorph is genetically destined to have higher amounts of fat than other body types and should not be expected to be able to create or maintain a very low percentage of fat. Also, a mesomorph would probably be heavier (TBW) than other body builds due to higher levels of lean body mass.

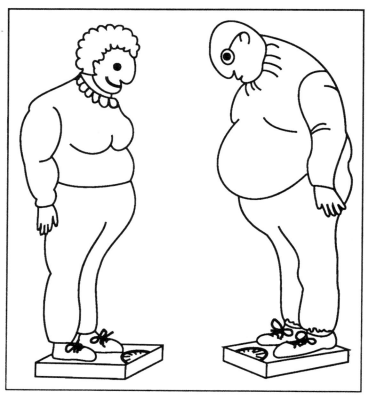

The bathroom scale is the most widely consulted scientific instrument in the world. Does it tell you what you really need to know?

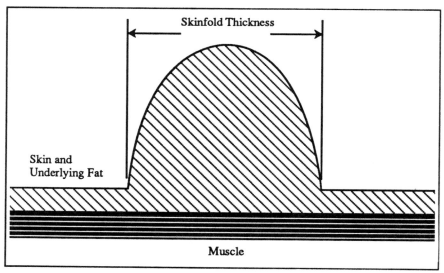

Most of the body's stored fat lies subcutaneously (under the skin). By measuring the thickness of skin and fat the total amount of fat in the body can be predicted. (See laboratory 3 dealing with Body Composition.)

Consequences of Obesity

When total percent body fat exceeds what is considered average or optimal, the amount of fat begins to have deleterious effects on health. Since **approximately 80 million people (about 40% of our population) can be considered obese, it is easy to understand why obesity is considered a medical problem in and of itself, in addition to causing or contributing to others.**

The list of dangers of being obese includes:

- ▶ diabetes
- ▶ hypertension
- ▶ heart disease
- ▶ stroke
- ▶ respiratory ailments
- ▶ kidney disease
- ▶ gall stones

- ▶ surgical risk
- ▶ pregnancy problems
- ▶ less resistance to infection
- ▶ longevity
- ▶ social discrimination
- ▶ psychological-emotional problems

In addition, where you are carrying excess body fat, *as your genetic fat pattern,* is significant. Scientific research has revealed two classic fat distribution patterns: android and gynoid, referring to male and female, respectively. The android pattern resembles an "apple shape," with the largest portion of weight around the middle. The gynoid pattern resembles a "pear shape," with most of the weight in the lower half. The apple shape is not restricted to males and the pear shape is not restricted to females. These fat storage tendencies are genetic.

Research studies have found that apple-shaped fat storage is accompanied by increased risk for high cholesterol, glucose intolerance (diabetes), and high blood pressure that may result from sodium retention. For pear-shaped fat storage, the most difficult problem may be the nonresponsiveness of these fat cells to diet and exercise. These fat cells cling to their fat content more tenaciously, therefore making diet and exercise efforts very frustrating. The risks of heart disease, diabetes, and hypertension do not appear to exist at the same level as with the apple shape fat storage pattern.

A *waist-to-hip ratio* is a method of assessing health risk relative to fat-pattern distribution. To compute this ratio, measure your waist (on skin, no clothing) and your hips (around the buttocks). Then divide the waist measurement by the hip measurement.

Ideally, your ratio will be less than 1.0. A reasonable ratio for women would be less than .90 and for men, less than .85. The goal is to keep this waist to hip ratio as low as possible by exercising and using a sensible low-fat diet.

Causes of Obesity

As mentioned previously, there is probably no one cause of obesity, but rather it is caused by an interaction of many factors. Recent research in the medical study of obesity supports the idea that **genetics** is the most important factor in the development of excess fatness. The fact that a fat person is not a glutton reflects this genetic control over how each individual processes the food that is eaten for the purpose of energy production and fat storage.

The major factor in developing obesity revolves around the food you eat, that is, the number of calories you consume. A **calorie** is an energy value of food. Different foods and varying amounts of food will enable the body to produce energy through a process called **metabolism.** Each individual requires a certain amount of calories (energy) just to live. This is called your **basal metabolic rate (BMR).** The basal metabolic rate is the amount of energy the body needs to carry on all its internal (basic) body functions. The mature adult needs 11 calories/lb to support the basal metabolism of the body. Thus, a person with greater mass requires more calories for basal metabolism than a lighter individual. If you consume more calories than you expend, it will result in the storage of unused calories as fat. The illustrations on page 37 show the relationship between consumption and expenditure of calories and the end result.

For some individuals, who may have both a genetic predisposition for obesity and a metabolic function that allows for greater fat storage, the number of calories they eat may not matter, since they will always store more as fat. Early determination of such a tendency is critical as is the need for dietary control and especially exercise.

Normal metabolic controls of energy may not exist in some people with genetic tendencies for obesity. Dr. Bernard Jeanrenaud at the University of Geneva has found that insulin is oversecreted at an early age in the genetically obese. This creates an insulin resistance in body cells that stimulates the production of more insulin. This disrupts the normal metabolism of blood glucose and inhibits the breakdown and use of fat for energy. This results in increased storage of fat in adipose tissue.

Kinds of Obesity

Recent findings indicate that there are at least two distinct types of obesity in human beings. One involves the number of fat cells and their consequent development, and the other involves the size of existing fat cells.

Childhood onset obesity (also called **early onset obesity**) reflects the number of fat cells that develop during pregnancy and early life of the child as a result of overfeeding. Once these cells are formed they may never disappear.

Adult onset obesity involves the increase in size of the existing fat cells as a result of overeating. This is often referred to as **creeping obesity,** that is, the gradual increase in fatness that seems to accompany increases in age.

The Role of Exercise

Weight control is a matter of controlling energy. It involves manipulating the variables that affect the energy equation. The two related sides of this equation involve the energy we consume in food (calories) and the energy we expend throughout the day largely for two purposes, resting metabolic requirements (RMR) and activity. When these two sides of the equation are equal, that is, calories in equal calories out, an isocaloric balance is created.

Energy expenditure includes several factors. The single largest expenditure of energy is the RMR (sometimes referred to as BMR, Basal Metabolic Requirements). This includes the energy used to maintain bodily functions in a resting state and is affected by body size (especially lean body mass), gender, and age.

Physical activity and exercise during the day also increase energy expenditure. The total caloric expenditure is determined by the length of time of activity/exercise and the effort required during that period of time.

Another factor that impacts the RMR is the energy required for the digestion, absorption, and transportation of nutrients after eating. This is referred to as the **thermic effect of eating** (TEE) or **dietary-induced thermogenesis** (DIT). The ingestion of food (eating) increases the energy expenditure by the body. Some food types contribute significantly to this process. Complex carbohydrates produce a high DIT compared to fats, which have a much lower effect (see chapter 4 for further discussion).

There are probably as many ways of dealing with weight control as there are people who are involved in that endeavor. Unfortunately, not enough people use exercise as one of those methods. Most use diet after diet after diet. Research over the years has shown a 95% failure rate with the "diet only" approach; that is, people just don't keep the weight off for more than a few months. This repeated cycle of weight loss followed by the regaining of weight is referred to as the "Yo-Yo syndrome." Each time the attempt is made to lose weight, it takes longer and less weight is lost and then the regain is faster with more of the weight being fat.

Interestingly, research completed over the past 10 years supports the fact that *the one factor that is most influential in preventing, reducing, and controlling obesity is exercise.*

The most effective weight loss is one that occurs over an extended period of time and involves a loss of about *1 lb per week.* This approach allows for a long-lasting modification of eating and activity habits. Exercise can make a significant contribution to the loss of body fat, especially when combined with a prudent choice of foods.

One lb of fat equals about 3,500 calories. Therefore, to lose 1 lb of fat you must perform enough activity to expend that much energy. This involves an unbelievable amount of physical exertion. However, when regular exercise is combined with caloric reduction, benefits are virtually guaranteed. For example, Golding and Zuti conducted a study in which three groups of women, all 20 to 40 lb overweight, were placed on a 500-calorie-per-day deficit for 16 weeks. One group was using a caloric restriction only approach, another group used an exercise only approach, and the third group combined caloric restriction plus increased activity. The results were as follows: The diet group loss was an average of 11.7 lb (9.3 lb fat and 2.4 lb lean body weight); the exercise group loss was an average of 10.6 lb (12.6 lb fat loss but a gain of 2 lb of lean body weight); and the combination group loss was an average of 12 lb (13 lb of fat and a 1 lb gain in lean body weight).

"The benefits of exercise in weight control extend far beyond the number of calories burned during the activity. In addition to raising the BMR for up to 15 hours afterward, exercise has been shown to have an appetite-suppressing effect, to enhance self-image and to reduce feelings of tension, anxiety and depression that prompt many people to overeat. Any kind of exercise is helpful that involves prolonged movement of the body's long muscles, as does walking, running, stair-climbing, swimming, cycling, skiing and skating."

In a study in California, 34 obese persons who had failed to maintain a weight loss on diet alone were started on a daily exercise program while consuming an unrestricted diet. All 11 who persisted for a year or more, most of them walking at least half an hour a day, lost weight—22 lb on the average—without dieting.

Exercise is also crucial to maintaining muscle tissue during a weight-loss program. A Chicago study among 32 college women who were 20% or more overweight showed that those who jogged three times a week and followed a reduced calorie diet lost more body fat and less lean muscle tissue than those who simply dieted.

However, Dr. Barry A. Franklin of Sinai Hospital in Detroit cautioned that passive exercise devices that "do the work for you" and spot-reducing gadgets are ineffective in producing weight loss or loss of selected fat deposits. "Unfortunately, the primary reduction often occurs in the exerciser's wallet," he said.[3]

Permanent and long-lasting "cures" for obesity have yet to be discovered. The combination of exercise and diet appears to be the most effective approach to taking off pounds and keeping them off. To lose fat you must expend more calories than you consume. A moderate reduction in calories is the key when accompanied by the best exercise for fat burning, which is aerobic. By using large muscle movements that elevate heart rate and the supply, delivery, and use of oxygen, aerobic exercise triggers muscle to burn more fat as fuel. This occurs predominately at lower levels of effort (intensity) and longer time periods (duration) of exercise, with 30 to 45 minutes being optimal. At higher levels of intensity (70% HR max and up), the energy being supplied for the exercise is produced in part anaerobically and more glycogen (sugar) and less fat is being burned.

When aerobic exercise is combined with strength training, the result seems to be more effective than with aerobic exercise alone. Running, cycling, swimming, dance exercise, and so on, do burn many calories, but when these are coupled with strength exercise, better body composition ratios are the result.

For example, in a recent study directed by Dr. Wayne Wescott at South Shore YMCA in Quincy, Massachusetts, the effects of two different exercise regimens were realized on body composition. Two groups of men and women used a recommended diet of 60% carbohydrates, 20% protein, and 20% fats. Both groups exercised 30 minutes each day, three days per week. However, one group performed 30 minutes of cycling on stationary bicycles while the other performed 15 minutes of cycling and 15 minutes of strength training. After eight weeks the aerobic exercisers lost an average of 3 lb of fat and a half pound of muscle. The aerobic/strength exercisers lost an average of 10 lb of fat and gained 2 lb of muscle for a 12-lb improvement.

Fat-Burning Guidelines

▶ Set reasonable and attainable goals—be realistic.

▶ Exercise aerobically at lower-intensity levels for 30 minutes or more at least three times per week.

▶ Consider resistance training as an adjunct to the aerobic exercise.

▶ Eat sensibly: adequate calories with emphasis on complex carbohydrate and less fat and sugar.

▶ Chart your progress with a caliper and tape measure rather than the bathroom scale.

A **positive calorie balance** exists when more calories are consumed than are expended. This situation is further complicated by the interaction of three major factors that cause creeping obesity: a reduction in basal metabolic rate as age increases; a tendency to decrease activity; and a tendency to maintain eating habits that are formed early in life. This combination has one end result—an increase in the amount of body fat and a usual increase in total body weight.

Attempting to lose body weight by either diet or exercise alone can be a discouraging process. However, when both exercise and diet are combined the end result is a **negative caloric balance** and its related weight loss. The following charts indicate the relationship between three elements of weight control—type of activity, duration of activity, and amount of caloric reduction. Through the interaction of these three elements the number of days required to lose a specified amount of weight can be determined. For example, if you wish to lose 10 lb and select walking as the mode of activity while decreasing your caloric intake by 400 calories per day, the expected result will occur in 54 days.

It must be remembered that the information on these charts is based on an individual weighing 154 lb and should not be considered to be absolute. For an individual weighing more than 154 lb, the energy cost for each activity will be greater; for an individual weighing less than 154 lb, the energy cost for each activity will be lower (see charts, pages 38–40).

The Set-Point Theory

A great deal of research over recent years supports the belief that there is a **set-point** for body weight and fatness that is automatically maintained by all our biochemical physiology. The theory is that without external influences the body strives to create and maintain a certain genetically determined weight and fatness. Some persons have a high setting or larger capacity for fat storage, whereas others have a low setting or smaller capacity for fat storage. Obviously, variations exist between the two extremes. The center for this set-point appears to be a section in the brain called the hypothalamus.

The set-points in animals and humans seem to change in response to two external factors: what you do (exercise) and what you eat. Sweet and fatty foods appear to drive the set-point higher. If the set-point theory is at all correct, exercise appears to be the best, if not the only, method for controlling a high set-point.

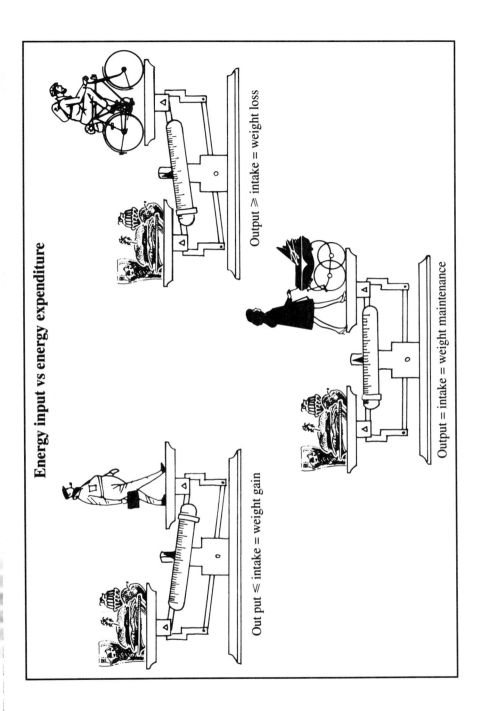

Energy input vs energy expenditure

Output ≥ intake = weight loss

Output = intake = weight maintenance

Out put ≤ intake = weight gain

37

Days Required to Lose 5 to 25 Lb by Walking* and Lowering Daily Calorie Intake

Minutes of Walking +	Reduction of Calories per Day (in kcal)	Days to Lose 5 Lb	Days to Lose 10 Lb	Days to Lose 15 Lb	Days to Lose 20 Lb	Days to Lose 25 Lb
30	400	27	54	81	108	135
30	600	20	40	60	80	100
30	800	16	32	48	64	80
30	1,000	13	26	39	52	65
45	400	23	46	69	92	115
45	600	18	36	54	72	90
45	800	14	28	42	56	70
45	1,000	12	24	36	48	60
60	400	21	42	63	84	105
60	600	16	32	48	64	80
60	800	13	26	39	52	65
60	1,000	11	22	33	44	55

*Walking briskly (3.5–4.0 mph), calculated at 5.2 Cal/minute.

Days Required to Lose 5 to 25 Lb by Bicycling* and Lowering Daily Calorie Intake

Minutes of Bicycling +	Reduction of Calories per Day (in kcal)	Days to Lose 5 Lb	Days to Lose 10 Lb	Days to Lose 15 Lb	Days to Lose 20 Lb	Days to Lose 25 Lb
30	400	25	50	75	100	125
30	600	19	38	57	76	95
30	800	17	34	51	68	85
30	1,000	13	26	39	52	65
45	400	22	44	66	88	110
45	600	17	34	51	68	85
45	800	14	28	42	56	70
45	1,000	12	24	36	48	60
60	400	19	38	57	76	95
60	600	15	30	45	60	75
60	800	13	26	39	52	65
60	1,000	11	22	33	44	55

*Bicycling calculated at 6.5 Cal/minute, at approximately 7 mph.

Days Required to Lose 5 to 25 Lb by
Swimming* and Lowering Daily Calorie Intake

Minutes of Swimming	+ Reduction of Calories per Day (in kcal)	Days to Lose 5 Lb	Days to Lose 10 Lb	Days to Lose 15 Lb	Days to Lose 20 Lb	Days to Lose 25 Lb
30	400	23	46	69	92	115
30	600	18	36	52	72	90
30	800	14	28	42	56	70
30	1,000	12	24	36	48	60
45	400	19	38	57	76	95
45	600	15	30	45	60	75
45	800	13	26	39	52	65
45	1,000	11	22	33	44	55
60	400	16	32	48	64	80
60	600	14	28	42	56	70
60	800	11	22	33	44	55
60	1,000	10	20	30	40	50

*Swimming at about 30 yards/minute calculated at 8.5 Cal/minute.

Days Required to Lose 5 to 25 Lb by
Stepping* and Lowering Daily Calorie Intake

Minutes of Stepping	+ Reduction of Calories per Day (in kcal)	Days to Lose 5 Lb	Days to Lose 10 Lb	Days to Lose 15 Lb	Days to Lose 20 Lb	Days to Lose 25 Lb
30	400	24	48	72	96	120
30	600	18	36	54	72	90
30	800	15	30	45	60	75
30	1,000	12	24	36	48	60
45	400	20	40	60	80	100
45	600	16	32	48	64	80
45	800	13	26	39	52	65
45	1,000	11	22	33	44	55
60	400	18	36	54	72	90
60	600	14	28	42	56	70
60	800	12	24	36	48	60
60	1,000	10	20	30	40	50

*Stepping up and down on a regular 7″ step at 25 steps/minute, calculated at 7.5 Cal/minute.

Days Required to Lose 5 to 25 Lb by Jogging* and Lowering Daily Calorie Intake

Minutes of + Jogging	Reduction of Calories per Day (in kcal)	Days to Lose 5 Lb	Days to Lose 10 Lb	Days to Lose 15 Lb	Days to Lose 20 Lb	Days to Lose 25 Lb
30	400	21	42	63	84	105
30	600	17	34	51	68	85
30	800	14	28	42	56	70
30	1,000	12	24	36	48	60
45	400	18	36	54	72	90
45	600	14	28	42	56	70
45	800	12	24	36	48	60
45	1,000	10	20	30	40	50
60	400	15	30	45	60	75
60	600	12	24	36	48	60
60	800	11	22	33	44	55
60	1,000	9	18	27	36	45

*Jogging—Alternate jogging and walking, calculated at 10.0 Cal/minute.

From *Exercise Equivalents of Foods: A Practical Guide for the Overweight* by Frank Konishi. Copyright © 1973 by Southern Illinois University Press. Reprinted by permission of Southern Illinois University Press.

Exercise and Appetite

Contrary to popular opinion, an increase in physical activity does not automatically create an increase in appetite. Conversely, an increase in physical activity does not automatically act as an appetite suppressant. The clear answer is that the appetite response to exercise is definitely individual in nature. However, intensity of exercise may play a key role in the desire for food. High-intensity exercise will selectively use more glycogen (carbohydrate) stores as the energy source and may thus affect blood sugar level at the end of exercise. Since blood sugar (blood glucose) may be somewhat low, the desire for food may be stimulated. Lower-intensity exercise appears to have a glycogen-sparing effect, since more fat is burned as fuel, and, therefore, may not increase appetite.

Studies have indicated, however, that energy intake and expenditure may not be balanced in the truly obese person. These people appear to eat in response to more varied environmental factors such as food availability (sight, sound, smell), time of the day, and social situations than do lean people. This can easily lead to creating a positive energy balance. Also, obese people do not seem to adjust appetite in response to varying levels of exercise, whereas lean people appear to adjust food intake to match energy expenditure.

A Lifelong Solution

To achieve permanent long-lasting weight control you must *integrate exercise into your life in such a manner as to effect a consistent body composition and weight throughout life.* This procedure requires a great deal of self-discipline and ever-constant awareness al change. At the same time exercise is infinitely more to your well-being than falling victim to sporadic diets or es that will not produce the desired results.

Summaryotyping is a subjective evaluation of body build. There are fjan ever-constant awareness of physical change. At the same time exercise is infinitely more valuable to your well-being than falling victim to sporadic diets or exercises that will not produce the desired results.

Summary

Somatotyping is a subjective evaluation of body build. There are three general classifications of body builds: endomorphs (stocky), mesomorphs (muscular), and ectomorphs (thin). Most people are mixtures of all three classifications with one classification usually dominant. Endomorphs are prone to obesity. Obesity is a significant problem to the general population. Height and weight charts may not be the best way to determine if you carry too much weight. The percentage of fat (overfat) may be a better way of determining excess weight, because body weight alone may indicate a high level of muscle development rather than fat. Obesity can contribute to a number of maladies, including high blood pressure, stroke, diabetes, and heart attack, as well as a reduced self-image.

▶ Obesity can best be controlled by a combination of diet and exercise.

▶ "Spot reducing" does not occur in response to exercising specific areas, such as sit-ups for the abdomen or leg lifts for the thighs.

▶ Exercise may alter body composition with little, if any, change in total body weight.

▶ One of the benefits of aerobic exercise is that it improves the ability to use fat as fuel; fit people are better fat burners.

▶ Body build (somatotype) and the distribution of body fat are more important than overall fat in relation to morbidity and mortality.

▶ Exercise tends to build muscles. Muscle is very metabolically active, burning more calories in resting metabolism than fat cells.

▶ Risks are associated with weight loss and with repeated diet failures—the yo-yo syndrome. Maintaining optimal body composition and weight is the key.

▶ Exercise does not automatically increase appetite and may decrease appetite for some people.

Diets: A Losing Effort

Not surprisingly, one of the most common four letter words in our society is DIET. Estimates reveal that as many as 25% of men and 50% of women are on a diet at any given time. The term "diet" has come to imply that in some way attempts are being made to lose weight by manipulating food consumption. Approximately $44 billion dollars was spent in 1991 on diets. Unfortunately, most people did not get their money's worth.

At best, the benefits of dieting are short term. At worst, research indicates that for the long term—dieting simply doesn't work. The most important reason why diets don't work for long-term weight loss lies in the fact that muscle is lost. Dieting actually worsens the most critical concern involved in weight gain—muscle loss—and this can result in weight gain as fat.

Typically, as we progress through our 20s, about one-half pound of muscle tissue is lost each year. Less muscle means a decrease in resting metabolic rate because muscle is very active tissue, even at rest. If this effect on metabolic rate is compounded by the effect of very low calorie dieting (VLCD) it is easy to see why the long-term effects can be disastrous. Even if we made no changes in the amount of calories we eat, weight will be gained because the caloric intake begins to exceed the body's caloric use. The result is a gain of a pound or more of fat each year.

The solution? Well, there is no cure but science has revealed the best control—exercise. With appropriate exercise, fat can be lost and lean weight (muscle) can be gained, allowing for optimal body composition values to be controlled for future years of life. Aerobic exercise combined with strength training produces the most favorable control. When you combine resistance training with aerobic exercise and sensible eating habits the result is increased lean body weight, decreases in fat weight, and improved fitness—you'll look better, feel better, function better.

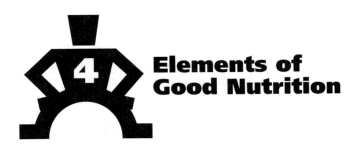

Elements of Good Nutrition

What you eat is one of two factors that will have the greatest influence on your well-being, excluding genetics. The other factor is exercise. To create the optimal benefit for well-being it is most prudent to maintain an exercise/diet connection. This connection provides its best benefit over a long time period, because the effects of both exercise and diet are accumulative. What exercise you do or what you eat on any single day will have little or no effect on your well-being for a lifetime. However, day by day, week by week, month by month, and year by year control of these factors will have definitive effects on quality and quantity of life. Diet, like exercise, can play a key role in weight control and general good health.

Americans seem to be obsessed with the control of body weight. It is estimated that as many as 80 million Americans are overweight and or obese to the point where it affects functional capacity adversely. At the same time we have available almost every conceivable diet imaginable: the Grapefruit diet, Stillman's diet, the Drinking Man's diet, Scarsdale diet, the Calories Don't Count diet, Slimfast diet, Optifast diet, and many more. Americans are dieting to the point where one out of four women and one out of five men are on some type of diet at any given time. Most diets do not keep excess weight and fat off on a permanent basis. Most of these VLCDs (very low calorie diets) create a loss of lean body weight (principally fluid and muscle) and not fat. Remember, VLCDs can drastically reduce your metabolic rate; therefore, it is not only unhealthy but it also can eventually lead to weight gain as fat rather than weight loss as fat. An end result of a VLCD can be **ketosis** (incomplete fat burn), which is caused by too few carbohydrates and can severely affect general body functions. To lose fat should be the goal and outcome of any weight-loss attempt. In some cases the goal is to prevent a weight gain as fat.

The desire to lose weight exceeds a rational concern for preventing the negative health consequences of obesity. We have arrived at a point where thinness has been equated with beauty. *Dieting (VLCD) is a very unhealthy behavior for two simple reasons:* (1) it doesn't work for the long haul; and (2) it leads to unhealthy situations such as a **yo-yo syndrome** (cycles of weight loss and gain), binge eating, and weight gain as fat.

Although Americans have available the most abundant and diverse food supply in the world much remains to be learned regarding control of this situation. A good diet provides all essential nutrients and enough energy to carry

43

on our daily activities, thus maintaining optimal health status. There are six classes of nutrients with only three providing energy (calories). These three are **proteins, carbohydrates,** and **fats.** The other three nutrients are **vitamins, minerals,** and **water.**

The most widely recommended approach to an adequate diet consists of combining groups of food that provide appropriate amounts of different nutrients, or a recommended daily allowance (RDA). The four major food groups that supply calories (energy) and nutrients (RDA) are:

Milk and Milk Products (Dairy)

Meat, Fish, Poultry, Beans

Vegetables and Fruits

Breads and Cereals (Grains)

Recently, the concept of a Food Pyramid has become the contemporary replacement for the basic four food groups. It portrays a fifth group—fats, oils, sweets—which appears at the top of the pyramid. The pyramid illustrates the relative amounts of the food groups that should form a sensible diet; most foods should come from the grain group and the fewest foods from the fat group.

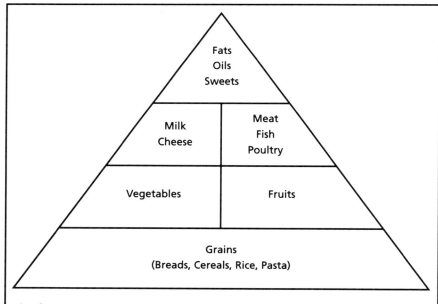

The food pyramid illustrates the food groups and the amounts of food that should be consumed from different groups.

Proteins

Proteins have always been considered the most important nutrient. They are needed for essential growth during youth and adolescence and are important for needed body repair by mature individuals. A lack of protein during the formative stages of life will result in diminished growth and vigor. It also leads to poor hair and skin condition and a slower healing process. Proteins contain twenty-two amino acids, which are broken down and used for the growth and repair process. Protein foods are classified as complete and incomplete. This refers to the number and proportions of amino acids present in a particular food. A protein such as egg whites and most red meats are complete proteins because of the presence of all necessary amino acids and the appropriate proportion of each. Vegetables, such as beans, provide some protein but are classified as incomplete protein. That is, the vegetable will not have all amino acids, and the amino acids would not be present in appropriate proportions. Most often, complete and incomplete proteins are included in the diet to satisfy needs. This would be different for a strict vegetarian and would present some distinct concerns relative to protein sources. Protein is not normally used as an energy source by cells except if carbohydrate and fat supplies are at low levels, a VLCD for example.

Typically, the American diet contains approximately 15% of all calories as protein. This appears to be adequate except perhaps for women who are pregnant, athletes who are trying to gain lean body mass (muscle), and adolescents who are pursuing athletics. The protein needs of these groups may be somewhat higher.

Protein does provide energy for cellular growth and repair. Its caloric content is 4 calories per gram (1/30 of an ounce).

Carbohydrates

Carbohydrates are our major sources of energy. They are usually available in abundance throughout the world and are often pleasant tasting "sweet" foodstuffs. Carbohydrates are classified as either simple (sugars) or complex. Sugar is the major source of sweet taste but carbohydrates are also found in starches present in many vegetables. The refining of carbohydrates causes a lower nutritive value. Refined carbohydrates, such as white table sugar (sucrose), have had the vitamins and minerals removed. Processed carbohydrate foods, such as flour for baking, are high in calories but low in vitamins and minerals.

This illustrates a concept known as *calorie density*. In this case the food provides energy (calories) but little, if any, vitamins, minerals, and fiber. If a food provides energy (calories) in addition to containing vitamins, minerals, and fiber, it is classified as *nutrient dense*.

Most of our carbohydrates are used on a daily basis but some is stored in the liver in the form of glycogen. The glycogen is secreted when the blood sugar is low and the muscles need additional energy. Carbohydrates are found in the bread and cereals group as well as in some fruits and vegetables. The major sources are sugar, bread, potatoes, pasta, and other white and yellow vegetables. The American diet contains about 50% carbohydrate intake and the figure is higher in some other cultures. The caloric yield of carbohydrates is, surprisingly, 4 calories per gram—the same as protein.

Carbohydrate is the most completely oxidized nutrient, yielding carbon dioxide and water during its breakdown into energy. As such, it has a very high dietary-induced thermogenesis, which means that complex carbohydrates contribute to increases in metabolism and, consequently, have little chance of being stored as fat. *Therefore, should you eat more complex carbohydrates? Absolutely!,* as much as 60% of your total daily caloric intake (and more, if you are a high-frequency, high-intensity exerciser) should be from carbohydrates.

Fats

Fat, or lipids are a key ingredient in the human diet. They serve as a source of energy and, when stored as adipose, cushion the major organs of the body. Almost half of all the fat in the body is a layer of fat beneath the skin to protect the body from extreme fluctuations in temperature. Fat provides protective padding beneath the kidneys as well as other vital organs. Fats slow down digestion, prompting the stomach to empty at a slower pace, which diminishes feelings of hunger. Fats often provide energy when the daily carbohydrate yield cannot provide needed energy. The primary source of fat is the milk and milk product group and meat and meat products. Foods such as butter, oils, whole milk, fatty meats, and ice cream are major sources of fat. Fats have a much higher yield of calories than proteins and carbohydrates (9 calories per gram) and are most easily stored as body fat if intake is excessive. The typical American diet includes about 40% of all calories from fat sources. The use of alcohol, with high calorie yield and little nutritive value, is also a contributor, although not a fat food. There also appears to be a relationship between excessive fat intake and high levels of cholesterol in the blood. High cholesterol levels have been identified as one of the major predisposing factors to heart disease and our diets should minimize foods that elevate cholesterol. Remember, *the fat you eat is the fat you wear*—in two places: in your arteries and under your skin.

Lipids (fats) are classified as either saturated or unsaturated (includes polyunsaturated and monounsaturated) based on the chemical formation. Saturated fats are solid at room temperature and are derived from animal sources: beef, lamb, pork, and butter, for example. There are only two saturated fat sources found in the plant kingdom: coconut and palm. These are very often used in commercial baking. Unsaturated fats are found in the plant kingdom. Sources would include corn oil, olive oil, safflower oil, cannola oil, and peanut oil. Although these contain the same number of calories per gram they are much less damaging to the cardiovascular system. These fats do not promote atherosclerosis and in addition to fatty oils found in fish (omega-3 oils) may help to reduce cholesterol.

There is little, if any, difference in the way normal weight subjects and obese subjects metabolize carbohydrates. The actual difference is the fat content of the diet. Virtually all fat calories are stored in fat cells waiting to be called on for use as energy. Fats have a very low *dietary-induced thermogenesis (DIT)*, so it is easy for the body to store them as fat. The bottom line is that simply reducing the total fat in a diet while continuing the same level of caloric intake can mean a slow weight loss. Combining the reduction of dietary fat with appropriate exercise provides the best control.

Vitamins

Vitamins are also essential to human life. They help the process by which proteins, carbohydrates, and fats are digested by the body. The best sources of vitamins are green, leafy vegetables. Beans, nuts, and whole grain cereals

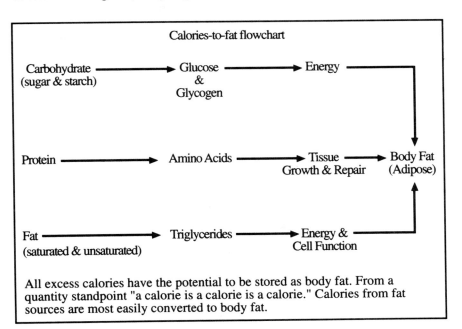

Calories-to-fat flowchart

All excess calories have the potential to be stored as body fat. From a quantity standpoint "a calorie is a calorie is a calorie." Calories from fat sources are most easily converted to body fat.

are also good sources of vitamins. Generally, an absence of vitamins will produce marked deficiencies or illness. Scurvy, the sailor's malady during the era of sailing ships, was attributable to the inability to store fresh fruits and a reliance on salted or cured meats. A balanced diet will probably enable you to receive all the necessary vitamins needed by your body. Many people take vitamin supplements without knowledge of which vitamins are truly deficient, which is costly and nonbeneficial. Many people "cover their bases" by the daily supplement, but they should be used sensibly.

Minerals

Minerals are also important for well-being. Calcium helps to build and maintain healthy teeth and bones and is found in milk and dairy products. Fluoride aids in strengthening bones and teeth. Seafoods and fluorinated water are its best source. Iodine, found in seafood and iodized salt, is necessary for the proper function of the thyroid gland (goiter prevention). Iron is stressed in most diets and is critical for the production of hemoglobin, which is the oxygen-carrying element in the blood. A lack of iron leads to anemia, characterized by a lack of vigor. Lean meats are the major source of iron. Potassium has received much concern in recent time. The daily banana as well as green, leafy vegetables promotes healthy skin and general well-being. Sodium regulates water in the body as well as blood pressure. An excess of sodium, particularly through salt intake, is thought to produce elevated blood pressure and excess weight through water retention.

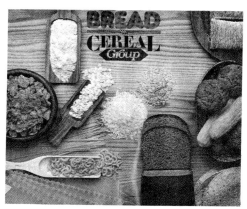

Bread and cereal group. (Source: *Food.* Home and Garden Bulletin Number 228. Prepared by Science and Education Administration, U.S. Department of Agriculture, 1979.)

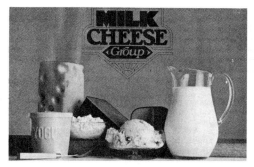

Milk and cheese group. (Source: *Food*. Home and Garden Bulletin Number 228. Prepared by Science and Education Administration, U.S. Department of Agriculture, 1979.)

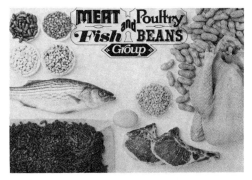

Meat, fish, poultry, and beans group. (Source: *Food*. Home and Garden Bulletin Number 228. Prepared by Science and Education Administration, U.S. Department of Agriculture, 1979, p. 9.)

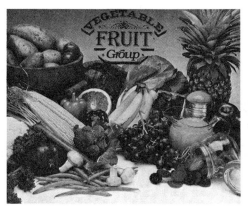

Vegetable and fruit group. (Source: *Food*. Home and Garden Bulletin Number 228. Prepared by Science and Education Administration, U.S. Department of Agriculture, 1979.)

Calorie Counter

Meat, Fish, Eggs	Size of Portion	Calories
Meat, fish, poultry lean-to-medium fat, averaged	1 serving (3 oz. cooked)	230
Liver	1 serving (3 oz. cooked)	180
Frankfurter	1 medium	125
Luncheon meat	2 medium slices (2 oz.)	165
Ham, boiled or baked	1 thin slice, 5 × 4″ (1 oz.)	85
Tuna or salmon, canned	3/8 cup (2 oz.)	105
Bacon, crisp	2 long slices (1/2 oz.)	100
Eggs	1 medium	75

Vegetables	Size of Portion	Calories
Green beans	1/2 cup, cooked	15
Carrots	1/2 cup, cooked	20
Beets	1/2 cup, cooked	35
Peas	1/2 cup, cooked	65
Lima beans	1/2 cup, cooked	75
Corn	1/2 cup, cooked	70
Potatoes, white	1 small potato, cooked	80
Potatoes, Mashed	1/2 cup	120
Potatoes, French Fried	6 pieces, 1/2 × 1/2 × 2″	120
Potatoes, sweet	1/2 medium potato, cooked	90
Raw carrot, tomato	1 small to medium	25
Celery	2 small stalks	5
Lettuce	1/4 medium head	10
Tossed salad, mixed vegetables	3/4 cup, without dressing	30

Dairy Foods	Size of Portion	Calories
Milk, whole	1 glass (8 oz.)	170
Milk, skim or buttermilk	1 glass (8 oz.)	85
Cheese, American or Swiss	1″ cube or medium slice (1 oz.)	110
Cheese, cottage creamed	2 tablespoons (1 oz.)	30
Butter	1 teaspoon or small pat	35
Cream, light, table	2 tablespoons	60
Half and Half	1/4 cup	80
Ice cream, vanilla	1/4 pint (1/2 cup)	150
Sherbet	1/2 cup	146

Bread and Cereals	Size of Portion	Calories
Bread, whole-grain or enriched	1 medium slice (4/5 oz.)	60
Cereal, cooked, whole-grain or enriched	1/2 cup	70
Cereal, ready-to-eat, whole-grained or enriched	1/2 cup	50
Rice or spaghetti	1/2 cup, cooked	105
Noodles	1/2 cup, cooked	55
Rolls, plain	1 small (1 oz.)	85
Rolls, sweet	1 medium (2 oz.)	180
Waffle	1 medium 4 1/2 × 5 1/2 × 1/2	215
Pancake	1 thin 4″ diameter	60
Crackers, plain or graham	2 medium	50

Calorie Counter—*Continued*

Pastries and Puddings	Size of Portion	Calories
Cookies, plain	2 small or 1 large	100
Cupcakes, iced	1 medium, 1 3/4" diameter	130
Cake, layer, plain icing	Med. piece, 1/6 6" cake	250–400
Cake, angel food or sponge	Small piece	115
Doughnut	1 medium	135
Pie, fruit	1/7 medium-size pie	300–350
Pie, custard type	1/7 medium-size pie	250–300

Fast-Foods Calorie Counts

The trouble with a scoop of Rocky Road ice cream is that it's a particularly rocky road to travel if you're on a strict diet. Still, the calorie count (204) might not be quite as high as you suspected—and it looks almost dietetic compared with the count (557) for McDonald's Big Mac. These and other fast-food calorie counts (approximate) below may or may not confirm your worst suspicions.

Arthur Treacher's Fish & Chips
An order of fish and chips (2 pieces of fish, 4 oz. of chips)—275.

Baskin-Robbins
One scoop (2 1/2 oz.) with sugar cone: Chocolate Fudge—229; French Vanilla—217; Rocky Road—204; Butter Pecan—195; Jomoca Almond Fudge—190; Chocolate Mint—189; Jomoca—182; Fresh Strawberry—168; Fresh Peach—165; Mango Sherbert—132; Banana Daiquiri Ice—129.

Burger King
The "Whopper"—606; the "Whaler"—744; bag of french fries (2 3/4 oz.)—214; large shake—332; hamburger—252; cheeseburger—305; hot dog—291.

Carvel
A standard 3 oz. cup of Vanilla ice cream—148; Chocolate ice cream—147; Sherbert—105; Vanilla, Chocolate or Coffee Thinny-Thin—55.5.

Chicken Delight
Average adult portion (1/2 chicken, 4 pieces)—625.

Colonel Sanders' Kentucky Fried Chicken
15-piece bucket—3300; drumstick—220; "3-piece special"—660; "dinner" (with 3 pieces of chicken, cole slaw, mashed potatoes, gravy, roll)—980.

Dairy Queen
Average banana split—547; "Super Brazier"—907; chicken snack—342.

Dunkin' Donuts
Hole-in-the-middle "cake" donuts; plain cake—240; plain honey-dipped—260; plain with white icing—265; plain with chocolate icing—235; chocolate cake—240; chocolate honey-dipped—250. "Yeast raised" donuts have jelly, custard or cream fillings: sugared—205; honey-dipped—225 (add 40–50 calories for filling).

Hardee's

"Huskee Deluxe"—525; "Huskee Junior"—475; fish sandwich—275; hot dog—265; apple turnover—290; average serving (2 oz.) french fries—155; milk shake (8 oz.)—320.

Howard Johnson's

25¢ cone: vanilla—186; chocolate—195; 35¢ cone: vanilla—247; chocolate—261. 45¢ cone: vanilla—370; chocolate—390; any flavor sherbert—136. (Hint for fried clam and pecan pie freaks: According to **The Brand-Name Calorie Counter:** 7 oz. pkg. Holo's frozen fried clams—357; 1/8 of a 2 lb. pecan pie—474.

Lum's

"The Ollie Burger" (5 1/2 oz. ground beef "with secret herbs and spices")—calories are a secret too but 5 1/2 oz. of broiled beef without a roll has 448. Average ounces in other Lum's portions, easily translated into calories with any pocket counter: fried onion rings— 5 1/2 oz.; hamburger—4 1/2 oz.

McDonald's

Egg McMuffin—312; Hamburger—249; Cheeseburger—304; Quarter Pounder with Cheese—521; Big Mac—557; Filet-of-Fish—406; french fries—215; Apple Pie—265; Chocolate Shake—317; Vanilla Shake—322; Strawberry Shake—315.

Taco Bell

One taco—159; tostada—188; order of frijoles—178; enchirito—418; burrito—319; "Bellburger"—243.

White Castle

Hamburger—157; serving of french fries—219; cheeseburger—198; fish sandwich—200; milk shake—213; serving onion rings—341; cinnamon roll—305; cherry roll—334.

Arby's

"Junior roast beef sandwich"—240; regular roast beef sandwich—429; turkey sandwich without Arby's dressing—337; with dressing—402; "ham 'n cheese—458; Arby's "Super" roast beef sandwich—705.

Sudol, Carol R.N., "Can You Have Your Diet & McDonald's Too?", **Community College Health Services,** E. D. Lovett, M.D., editor, Mt. View, Calif., Feb. 1978, Vol. 8, No. 6, p. 3.

The Good Diet

In addition to weight control, can sensible eating increase health status? Very definitely! One way in which this can happen is due to the effect of food and its nutrients on the immune system. To bolster the immune system with nutrients may mean fewer colds, viruses, and even cancers and quicker recovery if you should become ill. Is nutrition a panacea for disease? No! But it can help. Some suggestions include: Cruciferous vegetables like broccoli, cabbage, and cauliflower may aid in reducing cancer risk because they contain indoles; foods high in vitamin C content, such as citrus fruits (green peppers included), act as antioxidants (retard aging) and enhance cellular immunity;

A Look at the Calories in Our Cocktails . . .

You might want to think of your beer, wine or cocktail glass as leaving the following "rings" . . .

Alcohol 61%
Protein 3%
Carbohydrate 36%

Beer
Calories per ounce: 12.5

Alcohol 80.5%
Protein 0.5%
Carbohydrate 19%

Wine
Calories per ounce: 24.3

Alcohol 100%

Hard liquor (80 proof)
Calories per ounce: 69.3

The above percentages represent not volume or weight, but rather the percentage of each beverage's total calories that come in the form of the nutrients listed.

	CALORIES	CARBO-HYDRATES (grams)	ALCOHOL (grams)
DISTILLED LIQUORS			
Liqueurs (cordials) — 1 cordial glass			
Anisette	75	7.0	7.0
Apricot brandy	65	6.0	6.0
Benedictine	70	6.6	6.6
Creme de menthe	67	6.0	7.0
Curacao	55	6.0	6.0
Brandy, California — 1 brandy glass	73	—	10.5
Brandy, cognac — 1 brandy glass	73	—	10.5
Cider, fermented — 6 oz.	71	1.8	9.4
Gin, rum, vodka, whiskey (rye/scotch) — 1 jigger			
80-proof	104	0.0	15.0
86-proof	112	0.0	16.2
90-proof	118	0.0	17.1
94-proof	124	0.0	17.9
100-proof	133	0.0	19.1
WINES — 1 wine glass			
Champagne, domestic	85	3.0	11.0
Dessert (18.8% alcohol by volume)	137	7.7	15.3
Madeira	105	1.0	15.0
Muscatel/port	158	14.0	15.0
Red, California	85	—	10.0
Sauterne, California	85	4.0	10.5
Sherry, dry, domestic	85	4.8	9.0
Table (12.2% alcohol by volume)	85	4.2	9.9
Vermouth, dry (French)	105	1.0	15.0
Vermouth, sweet (Italian)	167	12.0	18.0
MALT LIQUORS (American) — 12 oz.			
Ale, mild	148	12.0	13.1
Beer, Budweiser	150	12.8	13.2
Beer, lite	96	2.8	12.1
Beer, Michelob	160	14.9	14.2
Beer, Natural Light	100	5.5	11.6
COCKTAILS			
Daiquiri — 1 cocktail	125	5.2	15.1
Eggnog (Christmas) — 4 oz.	335	18.0	15.0
Gin rickey — 8 oz.	150	1.3	21.0
Manhattan — 1 cocktail	165	7.9	19.2
Martini — 1 cocktail	140	0.3	18.5
Mint julep — 10 oz.	212	2.7	29.2
Old-fashioned — 4 oz.	180	3.5	24.0
Planters punch — 4 oz.	175	7.9	21.5
Rum sour — 4 oz.	165	—	21.5
Tom collins — 10 oz.	180	9.0	21.5
Whiskey sour — 1 cocktail	138	7.7	—
MIXERS — 4 oz.			
Club soda	0	0.0	0
Tonic water	44	11.0	0
Bitter lemon	64	14.1	0
Collins mixer	42	10.8	0
Ginger ale	45	11.3	0
Cola	43	12.0	0
Orange juice	28	6.0	0
Tomato juice	24	5.2	0

Glass Sizes: Cordial ⅔ oz.; brandy 1 oz.; jigger 1½ oz.; sherry 2 oz.; cocktail 3 oz.; wine 4 oz.; champagne 5 oz.

Source: From FOOD VALUES OF PORTIONS COMMONLY USED, Thirteenth Edition, Revised by Jean A. T. Pennington and Helen Nichols Church. Copyright © 1980 by Helen Nichols Church, B.S. and Jean A. T. Pennington, Ph.D., R.D. Reprinted by permission of HarperCollins Publishers.

fish (specifically those found in cold waters) rich in omega-3 fatty acids may aid in reducing cancer and heart disease risk; zinc, a mineral vital for the immune system, can be found in oysters, most other seafoods, and meats as well as a variety of legumes; and vitamins A and E serve as antioxidants and, therefore, make cells more resistant to cancer.

Food products from animal sources contain cholesterol with egg yolks as a highly concentrated source. Organ meats (liver, kidney, etc.) are also high in cholesterol and should be eaten sparingly. In addition, vegetable oils such as cottonseed or soybean are preferable to butter. Generally, meats should be broiled and served without heavy sauces. Heavy salad oils should also be avoided. Dessert choices should be fruit or sherbet rather than ice cream or whipped cream desserts. (To evaluate caloric intake and expenditure, see Laboratory 6.)

Eating Problems

Our society seems to be preoccupied with "thinness." Unrealistic expectations become commonplace and can drive one toward disordered eating patterns. Our cultural and societal messages about appearance create tremendous pressure on one to try and conform to an "ideal" weight, and/or physique. This expectation can lead to unhealthy eating patterns such as **bulimia** and **anorexia nervosa.** The pursuit of "the perfect fitness appearance" can contribute to these problems.

Anorexia nervosa is a "body image" problem. Some people believe they are or look "too fat" and severely restrict food intake to the point where hospitalization may be necessary.

Bulimia involves an attempt at controlling caloric intake by engaging in frequent episodes of binging (eating large volumes of food) and purging (self-induced vomiting, fasting, or laxative abuse).

Disorders of eating behaviors can also include chronic dieting and regain of weight (yo-yo syndrome), following VLCDs and pursuing body weight and food as an obsession.

The key to fitness and body weight control is to pursue healthful behaviors, which include regulation of exercise and diet, allowing for optimal function.

General Guidelines for a Fat-Modified Diet to Reduce the Risk of Heart Attack*

Every day, select foods from each of the basic food groups in lists 1 to 5.

Food Group	Nutrient Supplies	Recommended	Avoid or Use Sparingly
1. Meat Poultry Fish Dried beans and peas Nuts Eggs	Protein Irons B complex vitamins Fats Cholesterol (from animal sources)	*Chicken, turkey, veal, fish in most of your meat meals for the week.* *Shellfish: clams, crab, lobster, oysters, scallops.* Use a 4-ounce serving as a substitute for meat. *Beef, lamb, pork, ham less frequently.* Choose lean ground meat and lean cuts of meat. Trim all visible fat before cooking. Bake, broil, roast or stew so that you can discard the fat which cooks out of the meat. *Nuts and dried beans and peas:* Kidney beans, lima beans, baked beans, lentils, chick peas (garbanzos), split peas are high in vegetable protein and may be used in place of meat occasionally. *Egg whites as desired.*	Duck, goose Shrimp is moderately high in cholesterol. Use a 4-ounce serving in a meat meal no more than once a week. Heavily marbled and fatty meats, spare ribs, mutton, frankfurters, sausages, fatty hamburgers, bacon, luncheon meats. Organ meats (liver, kidney, heart, sweetbreads) are very high in cholesterol. Since liver is very rich in vitamins and iron, it should not be eliminated from the diet completely. Use a 4-ounce serving in a meat meal no more than once a week. Egg yolks: limit to 3 per week, including eggs used in cooking. Cakes, batters, sauces, and other foods containing egg yolks.

*From *Heartbook* by American Heart Association. Copyright © 1980 by American Heart Association. Used by permission of the publisher, Dutton, an imprint of New American Library, a division of Penguin Books USA Inc.

General Guidelines for a Fat-Modified Diet   *Continued*

Food Group	Nutrient Supplies	Recommended	Avoid or Use Sparingly
2. Vegetables and Fruits (Fresh, frozen, or canned)	Vitamins A & C Minerals Fiber Carbohydrates	*One serving should be a source of vitamin C:* Broccoli, cabbage (raw), tomatoes. Berries, cantaloupe, grapefruit (or juice), mango, melon, orange (or juice), papaya, strawberries, tangerines. *One serving should be a source of vitamin A— dark green leafy or yellow vegetables, or yellow fruits:* Broccoli, carrots, chard, chicory, escarole, greens (beet, collard, dandelion, mustard, turnip), kale, peas, rutabagas, spinach, string beans, sweet potatoes and yams, watercress, winter squash, yellow corn. Apricots, cantaloupe, mango, papaya. Other vegetables and fruits are also very nutritious; they should be eaten in salads, main dishes, snacks, and desserts, in addition to the recommended daily allowances of high vitamin A and C vegetables and fruits.	If you must limit your calories, use vegetables such as potatoes, corn, and lima beans sparingly. To add variety to your diet, one serving (½ cup) of any one of these may be substituted for one serving of bread or cereals.

General Guidelines for a Fat-Modified Diet *Continued*

Food Group	Nutrient Supplies	Recommended	Avoid or Use Sparingly
3. Bread and cereals (whole grain, enriched, or restored)	Iron Niacin Carbohydrates Protein Fiber	*Breads made with a minimum of saturated fat:* White enriched (including raisin bread), whole wheat, English muffins, French bread, Italian bread, oatmeal bread, pumpernickel, rye bread. Biscuits, muffins, and griddle cakes made at home, using an allowed liquid oil as shortening. Cereal (hot and cold), rice, melba toast, matzo, pretzels. Pasta: macaroni, noodles (except egg noodles), spaghetti.	Butter rolls, commercial biscuits, muffins, donuts, sweet rolls, cakes, crackers, egg bread, cheese bread, commercial mixes containing dried eggs and whole milk.
4. Milk products	Vitamins A & D Protein B vitamins Calcium Phosphorus Carbohydrates	*Milk products that are low in dairy fats:* Fortified skimmed (non-fat) milk and fortified skimmed milk powder, low-fat milk. The label on the container should show that the milk is fortified with Vitamins A and D. The word "fortified" alone is not enough. Buttermilk made from skimmed milk, yogurt made from skimmed milk, canned evaporated skimmed milk, cocoa made with low-fat milk.	*Whole milk and whole milk products:* Chocolate milk, canned whole milk, ice cream, all creams including sour, half-and-half, and whipped; whole milk yogurt. Non-dairy cream substitutes (usually these contain coconut oil, which is very high in saturated fat). Cheese made from cream or whole milk. Butter.

General Guidelines for a Fat-Modified Diet *Continued*

Food Group	Nutrient Supplies	Recommended	Avoid or Use Sparingly
		Cheese made from skimmed or partially skimmed milk, such as cottage cheese, creamed or uncreamed (uncreamed is preferable), farmer's, baker's, or hoop cheese, mozzarella and sapsago cheeses. Processed modified fat cheeses (skimmed milk and polyunsaturated fat).	
5. Fats and oils (Polyunsaturated)	Essential fatty acids Vitamins A & D	*Margarines, liquid oil shortenings, salad dressings and mayonnaise containing any of these polyunsaturated vegetable oils:* Corn oil, cottonseed oil, safflower oil, sesame seed oil, soybean oil, sunflower seed oil. Margarines and other products high in polyunsaturates can usually be identified by the label, which lists a recommended liquid vegetable oil as the first ingredient, and one or more partially hydrogenated vegetable oils as additional ingredients. Diet margarines are low in calories because they are low in fat. Therefore it takes twice as much diet margarine to supply the polyunsaturates contained in a recommended margarine.	*Solid fats and shortenings:* Butter, lard, salt pork fat, meat fat, completely hydrogenated margarines and vegetable shortenings, products containing coconut oil. Peanut oil and olive oil may be used occasionally for flavor, but they are low in polyunsaturates and do not take the place of the recommended oils.

Summary

The old expression "you are what you eat" may be more true than ever expected. It has become obvious that diet is extremely important in preventing and combating disease processes. Much research supports the concept that a very low fat diet, in conjunction with exercise, may actually reduce existing plaque buildup in arteries. Remember, it is a two-sided coin where diet is concerned—not only what you eat but also how much.

Care must be taken with vitamin and/or mineral supplementation. Toxicity (physiological problems) can be created by overdosing with vitamins and minerals. Consult a reliable source of information for vitamin/mineral overdosing.

Three questions are important relative to dietary selections and, therefore, impact on health status:

1. Are the majority of foods I have chosen good sources of complex carbohydrates?

2. Have I included good sources of vitamins A, C, and E in my daily meals?

3. Have I included a good source of protein that is low in fat?

Try to use the following approximate breakdown of daily calories for a "calorie meal plan":

▶ Breakfast　　25–30%

▶ Lunch　　　 20–25%

▶ Dinner　　　30–35%

▶ Snacks　　　 5–10%

"Healthy" Weight

Our culture provides the perfect recipe for the development of problems associated with nutritional practices: an abundant food supply and a sedentary life-style. When we combine these with an unrealistic standard of thinness by which people are judged, it is easy to understand why dieting is probably the number one nutrition pursuit.

Over the last 10 years, the advice offered in the Dietary Guidelines for Americans published by the U.S. Department of Agriculture has ranged from maintaining an "ideal weight," then a "desirable weight," and most recently a "healthy weight." This "healthy weight" is recognized as the point at which there is little if any risk for weight/fat-related diseases. Three questions will aid in determining "healthy weight" and any need for change: (1) Are you within an acceptable weight range for your age, height, and somatotype? (2) Is your waist-to-hip ratio below the recommended values of .90 for women and .85 for men? and (3) Do you have an existing condition that would benefit from weight reduction, such as diabetes or hypertension?

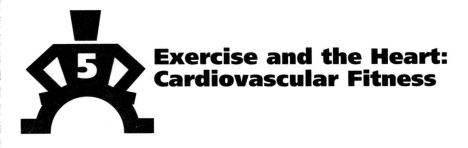

Exercise and the Heart: Cardiovascular Fitness

The Heart and Cardiovascular Disease

Cardiovascular diseases (CVD) are the major causes of death in the United States. They represent approximately 50% of disease-related deaths. Heart attacks strike more than one million Americans each year, while the remaining CVD deaths are attributable to conditions like hypertensive disease (high blood pressure), rheumatic heart disease, and congenital heart disease.

Heart diseases have generally been thought to affect older members of the population and yet a frightening new trend has emerged that indicates a striking increase in heart attacks among the young and middle-aged adult. The trend for heart attacks among younger men has been rising steadily for two decades. For men between 25 and 44, the coronary death rate has gone up 14%—from 46 to 52 per 100,000 since 1950. This year, approximately 31% of Americans who will die from coronaries will be under 65, victims of what public health officials call "premature" heart disease. Statistics show that of all deaths due to CVD, more than 20% are younger than 65 years of age. In men between 40 and 60 years of age 40%, of the deaths are due to some form of CVD called coronary heart disease (CHD).

Cardiovascular disease occurs when a part of the cardio (heart) vascular (blood vessels) system can no longer function adequately enough to deliver blood throughout the body. The failure of the cardiovascular system can be due to many reasons. It is characteristically caused by a reduction in the open space (lumen) through which blood flows to the heart muscle (myocardium) and supplies it with blood and oxygen.

The heart is a four-chambered double pump that beats roughly 100,000 times a day to pump blood through 60,000 miles of blood vessels. The right side of the heart receives blood after it has been returned with waste products (carbon dioxide) from the body and sends the blood to the lungs. The lungs cleanse the blood of the carbon dioxide and provide oxygen from respiration. The oxygenated blood is returned to the left side of the heart where it is pumped out to the body. The number of times the heart pumps per minute will vary between 60 and 95 in normal hearts.

Atherosclerosis is a progressively slow disease that has an onset early in life and continues to narrow the cross section of the arteries by increasing the fat buildup on the lining of the arteries. **Lesions** (sores) develop in the walls of the coronary arteries encouraging this fat buildup called **plaque.** Over time, blood flow is reduced to the myocardium, resulting in **ischemia** (lack of oxygen). The buildup of fatty materials on the inner lining of the blood vessels also diminishes the ability of the arteries to expand and contract. The blood does not move as easily through the narrowed arteries, which may enable a clot to occur, thus depriving the heart of life-giving blood. Atherosclerosis will also cause the heart muscle to work harder to get the blood through the arteries, thus increasing blood pressure.

Heart attack is not usually a surprise. The predisposing causes of the disease such as atherosclerosis have been building up for years, but the victim has been unaware of the process. A blood clot or thrombus forms in a narrowed artery causing a **coronary thrombosis,** which may completely eliminate the flow of blood to the heart. The stoppage of blood to the heart results in a **myocardial infarction,** which is the death of heart tissue and subsequent scar formation. The question of a victim surviving a heart attack may depend on the extent of the myocardial infarction and whether **coronary collateral circulation** is present. Coronary collateral circulation provides a series of small blood vessels to carry blood when the larger coronary arteries are blocked. These vessels may be working prior to an attack as more coronary vessels become clogged. It is thought that exercise plays a key role in creating these collateral arteries and that trained people have a better chance of surviving a heart attack because of the additional blood flow. The majority of people who die from myocardial infarction die within two hours, usually because the heart beats uncontrollably, out of rhythm (ventricular fibrillation). The normal heart rate is controlled by special heart cells in the sinus node (pacemaker). Electrical impulses travel to the heart's working muscle cells, causing them to contract and pump blood. The normal heart rate varies between 60 and 95. A heart rate under 60 is called bradycardia and could be evidence of excellent training or of disease. Heart rates above 100 are called tachycardia and often indicate illness.

It is also possible to have a heart attack caused by an **embolus,** which is a wandering clot. This clot may become lodged in a narrow arterial channel and block blood flow.

The victim of a heart attack may have had some early warning from **angina pectoris.** Chest pains develop during a heart attack, but they often occur at times prior to the actual attack. A lack of oxygen caused by diminished blood flow can be mild or oppressive as in a heart attack. The symptoms should not be ignored. Pain usually occurs during physical exertion and may be absent at rest.

Stroke occurs when the brain does not receive enough oxygen. A common cause of stroke is a clot or thrombus in cerebral arteries. An embolus can also cause a stroke. A stroke may be induced by the breaking of a blood vessel supplying the brain, which distends and damages brain tissue. Stroke can cause difficulty in walking, paralysis, and loss of memory. The extent of the impairment will depend on how much damage is caused to the brain tissue. Cerebral hemorrhage (stroke) is often associated with high blood pressure.

Multiple Risk Theory

Presently, a *multiple risk theory* concerning the development of cardiovascular disease and atherosclerosis is widely accepted. Some of the risk factors seem to have a stronger association with atherosclerosis and cardiovascular disease than others. These are called primary risk factors and include:

▶ High cholesterol level

▶ Hypertension (high blood pressure)

▶ Cigarette smoking

Other factors that are associated, but less strongly, are called secondary risk factors. These include:

▶ Obesity	▶ Stress (psychological)
▶ Inactivity	▶ Family history (heredity)
▶ Gender	▶ Diabetes
▶ Age	

Death Rates

No. 110. Death Rates by Sex, Age, and Selected Causes: 1980

[Deaths per 100,000 resident population enumerated as of April 1. Causes of death classified according to ninth revision of the *International Classification of Diseases*]

Cause of Death	Total[1]	Male					Total[1]	Female				
		Total[1]	15–24 years	25–44 years	45–64 years	65 yrs. and over		Total[1]	15–24 years	25–44 years	45–64 years	65 yrs. and over
All causes[2]	878.3	976.9	172.3	238.0	1,270.0	6,387.9	785.3	57.5	110.2	670.9	4,484.1
Diseases of heart	336.0	368.6	3.7	34.6	505.3	2,778.6	305.1	2.1	11.9	177.3	2,027.5
Malignant neoplasms	183.9	205.3	7.8	25.8	348.0	1,371.6	163.6	4.8	30.1	265.8	767.8
Cerebrovascular diseases	75.1	63.6	1.1	5.1	50.0	557.0	86.1	.8	5.0	39.9	584.0
Accidents and adverse effects	46.7	67.4	96.7	68.6	61.9	124.4	27.1	26.0	17.3	21.6	78.9
Chronic obstructive pulmonary diseases[3]	24.7	35.1	.4	1.0	35.0	297.9	15.0	.3	.9	17.6	84.5
Pneumonia and influenza	24.1	25.1	.8	2.9	17.8	212.5	23.2	.8	1.8	8.7	154.9

64

Diabetes mellitus	15.4	13.0	.3	2.7	18.2	92.8	17.6	.3	2.0	17.7	102.7
Chronic liver disease and cirrhosis	13.5	18.0	.3	10.3	50.5	56.0	9.3	.3	5.0	23.2	24.6
Atherosclerosis	13.0	10.5	—	.1	4.0	104.0	15.3	—	.1	2.0	113.9
Suicide	11.9	18.6	20.2	24.0	23.7	35.0	5.5	4.3	7.7	8.9	6.1
Certain conditions originating in the perinatal period	10.1	11.9	(X)	(X)	(X)	(X)	8.4	(X)	(X)	(X)	(X)
Homicide and legal intervention	10.7	17.3	24.5	29.4	15.4	8.9	4.5	6.6	6.4	3.4	3.3
Nephritis, nephrotic syndrome and nephrosis	7.4	7.8	.2	1.2	7.1	63.6	7.0	(Z)	.7	5.5	42.1

— Represents zero.   X Not applicable.   Z Less than .05.

1. Includes persons under 15 years old, not shown separately.

2. Includes other causes, not shown separately.

3. Includes allied conditions.

Source: U.S. National Center for Health Statistics, *Vital Statistics of the United States*, annual, and unpublished data.

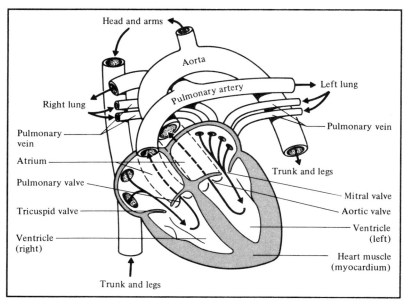

The human heart, like the heart in all mammals, has four chambers. Two of these chambers (one atrium and one ventricle) perform systemic circulation. The two remaining chambers carry out pulmonary circulation. There is a wall between the chambers (the septum), which prevents oxygenated blood from mixing with deoxygenated blood. Valves between the atria and ventricles prevent backward flow when the heart contracts. (Reprinted with permission of Macmillan Publishing Company from *Health Now* by Stephen E. Gray and Hollis Matson. Copyright © 1976 by Macmillan Publishing Company)

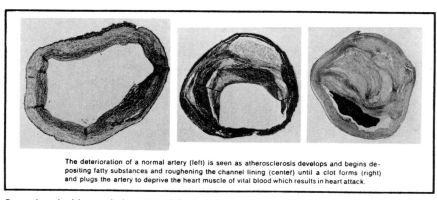

The deterioration of a normal artery (left) is seen as atherosclerosis develops and begins depositing fatty substances and roughening the channel lining (center) until a clot forms (right) and plugs the artery to deprive the heart muscle of vital blood which results in heart attack.

Reproduced with permission. Copyright American Heart Association.

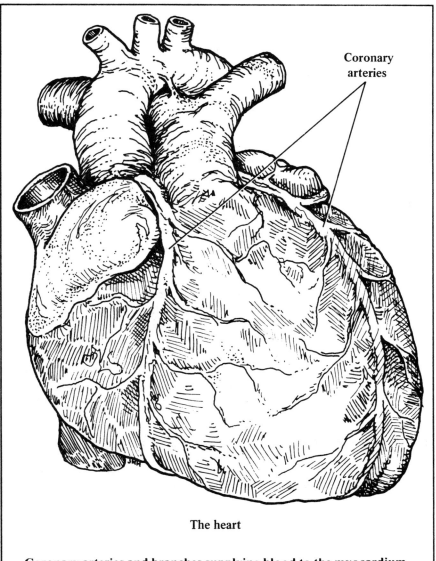

Coronary
arteries

The heart

Coronary arteries and branches supplying blood to the myocardium.

Uncontrollable Factors Related to Heart Disease

Age—Generally, the older a person gets, the more susceptible he or she becomes to cardiovascular disease. The risk increases significantly above fifty years of age, although we continue to see an increase in debilitating heart attacks striking people as young as 30 or 40. One in four victims of heart attack deaths is under the age of 65. Stroke, which is considered to be a disease of the older person, strikes people at an increasingly younger age. One in six of all stroke deaths occurs under the age of 65. The specific cause can probably be attributed to a number of contributing factors, including the deterioration of the cardiovascular system with age.

Sex—Men have more cardiovascular disease than women. They encounter difficulty earlier in life and die more often from the disease. Such problems as high blood pressure strike men as much as an average of 10 years earlier than women. One theory is that the female hormone estrogen may protect the female against heart attack and related diseases, as the incidence increases significantly after menopause, which brings about a decrease in estrogen production. The entrance of women into decision-making and stressful positions during the last decade is being accompanied by increases in heart disease among women. Stress is thought to be a factor in the increase.

Heredity—We inherit many characteristics from our parents and grandparents. Evidently, we may inherit a tendency toward susceptibility to disease in the circulatory system. Although there is no direct evidence that heart attack and stroke or the process of atherosclerosis is hereditary, the incidence is higher in some families than others. The susceptibility to a number of the factors that increase risk are probably inherited. Certain families inherit specific tendencies to cardiovascular disease and have limited life expectancy as a result.

Heart Disease Risk Factors That You Can Control

The factors related to heart disease that we can control are very important and may be remembered by the acronym CHOSE.

C—cholesterol (as related to saturated fat intake)

H—high blood pressure

O—obesity

S—smoking and stress

E—exercise

Cholesterol—An elevation of this lipid (blood fat) is positively correlated with coronary heart disease (CHD). The risk decreases when the level of total serum cholesterol is below 200 mg/100 ml of blood and increases proportionally above this level. It is important to understand that two types of lipids form cholesterol in the blood. These are high-density lipids (HDLs) and low density lipids (LDLs). The low-density lipids are responsible for the formation of plaque (fatty deposits) on the interior walls of the arteries, thus decreasing blood flow and resulting oxygen supply. This is critical in the coronary and cerebral arteries. The high-density lipids do not become encrusted on the arterial lining and may actually help remove circulating LDLs. In addition to lowering the total cholesterol level, the HDL cholesterol level has become a good indication of developing atherosclerotic plaquing. In adult men HDL levels should be above 45% and in women above 55%.

The body manufactures its own cholesterol in addition to receiving it in the diet. Cholesterol may be metabolized at an increased rate with regular exercise. Studies have shown that only about 30% of the dietary intake of cholesterol is absorbed. The liver is responsible for producing body cholesterol and its production level depends on the amount of fat that enters the diet. Engorging large amounts of food, a sedentary life-style, and cigarette smoking can cause elevated blood cholesterol. Evidence also indicates that plasma **triglycerides,** another lipid, may be a contributor to CHD. The end result of the accumulation of these blood lipids is a cardiovascular problem called atherosclerosis.

A change in the diet to reduce saturated fats that are found in fatty meats, butter, cheese, and milk is often recommended in addition to measurement of the plasma lipids as part of a routine physical examination. Exercise will also play a critical part in the control of the blood lipids.

High Blood Pressure (Hypertension)—Blood pressure is the force of the blood against the arterial walls. The force is generated by the heart as it pumps to keep blood moving through the arteries. The artery walls are muscular and elastic. The blood pressure increases as the heart pumps and decreases as the heart relaxes.

Blood pressure is elevated in many people. The cause is not specifically known but the high level could be caused by change in body chemistry (due to a defect in an organ such as a kidney), emotional stress, and possible hereditary implication. High blood pressure causes the heart to overwork. The elevation of blood pressure against the arterial walls causes the heart to pump more often and it will eventually weaken. The arterial walls will eventually lose their elasticity, thus contributing to **arteriosclerosis (hardening of the arteries).** Risk of premature cardiovascular disease and death rise sharply with increase in blood pressure. The vessels may not be able to deliver enough oxygen to the body. A blood pressure reading of 120/80 is thought to be normal. However, upper level readings **(systolic)** between 100 and 140 are also thought to be normal as well as lower level readings **(diastolic)** of 60 to 90. Some symptoms of high blood pressure include dizziness, lightheadedness, fatigue, shortness of breath, and headaches.

Medicines are very effective in lowering blood pressure to acceptable limits and maintaining those limits. Change in diet to lower fat levels, and cessation of smoking are also important considerations.

Obesity—Additional weight above the person's normal weight is considered to be harmful, because it causes the heart to work harder to provide oxygen for the increased body mass. Thus, the heart will enlarge, pump more times per day, and the individual will tire more readily.

Normal weight is adjudged as meeting standards set in traditional height and weight charts. Overweight is generally described as being 10% above the person's optimal (best) weight. Obesity is described as 20% above the optimal weight. These standards are misleading and may not reflect the true nature of weight difficulty.

The percentage of body fat as described in chapter 3 may be the most important indicator of weight problems, as the published ideal weight charts do not reflect variability of body build and body density.

Smoking—The relationship between smoking and heart disease was illuminated in the Surgeon General's report of 1964. Up until then, smoking was thought to be most harmful to the lungs. The report reinforced this concept but also indicated the serious consequences of smoking as it relates to heart disease.

> "Smoking and nicotine administration cause acute cardiovascular effects similar to those induced by stimulation of the autonomic nervous system, but these effects do not account well for the observed association between cigarette smoking and coronary disease. It is established that male cigarette smokers have a higher death rate from coronary disease than non-smoking males. Other factors such as high blood pressure, high serum cholesterol and excessive obesity are also known to be associated with an unusually high death rate from heart disease."[4]

Evidence established since the report indicates that female cigarette smokers are suffering heart attack deaths in a similar manner as men.

The 1979 Report of the Surgeon General on Smoking and Health identifies smoking as causally related to coronary heart disease for both sexes in the United States, and cigarette smoking as a *major independent risk factor for the development of fatal and nonfatal myocardial infarction.*

Experimental studies indicate carbon monoxide from smoking causes damage to the inner lining of the blood vessels, enabling fluids and fats to form in the wall of the blood vessels. Nicotine also elevates blood cholesterol. Arterial blood pressure is increased by nicotine and the carbon monoxide present in the blood decreases the available oxygen. This causes the heart muscle to work harder. The arterial walls also contract, which elevates the blood pressure and makes the heart beat faster. In addition, carbon monoxide and nicotine cause the possibility of **ventricular fibrillation,** that is, the heart beating wildly out of rhythm. Ventricular fibrillation usually occurs when there is an ischemia or lack of oxygen due to narrowing of the coronary arteries. The supposition is that sudden, unexpected deaths could be due to this condition.

Smoking has also been found to increase the risk of lung cancer, emphysema, and chronic bronchitis and contributes to a higher rate of miscarriage to women who smoke. Women's lung cancer rates have now surpassed breast cancer as the leading cause of death in women.

As stated in *Cancer Facts & Figures—1992,* the American Cancer Society estimates that cigarette smoking is responsible for 90% of lung cancer deaths among men and 79% among women—87% overall. This reflects the fact, that in the past, more men than women smoked and smoked more heavily. However, the gap between the numbers of men and women smoking has been narrowing. Those who smoke two or more packs of cigarettes a day have lung cancer mortality rates 15 to 25 times greater than nonsmokers.

Smoking is also associated with cancers of the mouth, pharynx, larynx, esophagus, pancreas, uterine cervix, kidney, and bladder. Smoking accounts for 30% of all cancer deaths, is a major cause of heart disease, and is associated with conditions ranging from colds and gastric ulcers to chronic bronchitis, emphysema, and cerebrovascular disease.

Smoking is the most preventable cause of death in our society. According to the World Health Organization, approximately 2.5 million people die worldwide each year as a result of smoking.

The more cigarettes a person smokes a day and the longer a person has smoked will increase his or her risk. A study done by the American Cancer Society indicates that a nonsmoker at age 25 can be expected to live until 73.6 years, pack-a-day smoker until 68.1, and a two pack-a-day smoker until 65.3. As few as 10 cigarettes per day can adversely affect endurance and cardiorespiratory function.

In September 1990, the Surgeon General released a report showing that people who quit smoking, regardless of age, live longer than people who continue to smoke. Smokers who quit before age 50 have one-half the risk of dying in the next 15 years compared with those who continue to smoke.

By 1987, more than 38 million Americans had quit smoking cigarettes, nearly half of all living adults who ever smoked. According to a 1989 Gallup survey, 57% of smokers 50 and older, 68% of smokers aged 18–29, and 67% of smokers aged 30–49 want to quit smoking.

The report states that "smoking cessation has major and immediate health benefits for men and women of all ages." Quitting smoking substantially decreases risks of lung, laryngeal, esophageal, oral, pancreatic, bladder, and cervical cancer. The benefits of cessation include risk reduction for other major diseases including coronary heart disease and cardiovascular disease.

Exercise—The level of exercise is of special importance in its relationship to heart disease. Vigorous, rational exercise can decrease the blood lipid levels in the bloodstream and increase the amount of blood available to the body by increasing the **stroke volume** of the heart. The stroke volume is the amount of blood that the heart pumps with each contraction. A heart muscle that is trained can pump more blood as it beats less times per minute. The amount of blood supplied to the cells per minute is the cardiac output. As the stroke volume increases due to training, less heart beats are needed to maintain the cardiac output, and the resting heart rate will drop as the stroke volume increases. The exercised heart will also have a better chance at surviving a heart attack through the development of coronary collateral blood vessels that enable blood to supply the heart despite a blockage in a main coronary artery.

Research studies of various occupations have found a lack of exercise to be correlated with development of the disease. Studies of bus drivers and conductors, postal clerks and telegraphers, and railroad clerks and railroad maintenance workers, among others, indicate higher incidence of CHD deaths among sedentary people than among active people. Current available evidence indicates that a physically inactive person has a higher risk of heart disease than a person who is physically active. In addition, evidence indicates that the chances of recovery from a heart attack are better for a person who has been physically active.

The American Heart Association has concluded, from existing evidence, that a lack of exercise is a risk factor in heart disease. Interestingly, "according to new findings presented to the American Heart Association, those who engage in vigorous exercise on a regular basis are likely to reduce in many ways the risk of developing heart disease. Studies of thousands of active individuals show that achieving physical fitness is associated with significant drops in weight, blood pressure, cholesterol levels and other factors associated with an increased risk of heart disease."[5]

Exercise also appears to elevate the level of **high-density lipoproteins** in the blood. These high-density lipoproteins seem to purge the blood of cholesterol. Certain types of these lipoproteins are higher in women and may be a factor in women being less prone to heart disease.

Studies of a large group of Harvard alumni (see illustration on page 73) showed that highly active people have significantly fewer heart attacks.

"Physicians who have studied the effects of exercise on heart function maintain that to derive significant benefits, exercisers should 'work up a sweat' for 20 minutes at least three times a week. Such a 'moderate' amount of activity would use up about 1,200 calories a week.

The continuing study of nearly 17,000 Harvard alumni has demonstrated that moderate physical exercise in adult life can significantly increase life expectancy."[6]

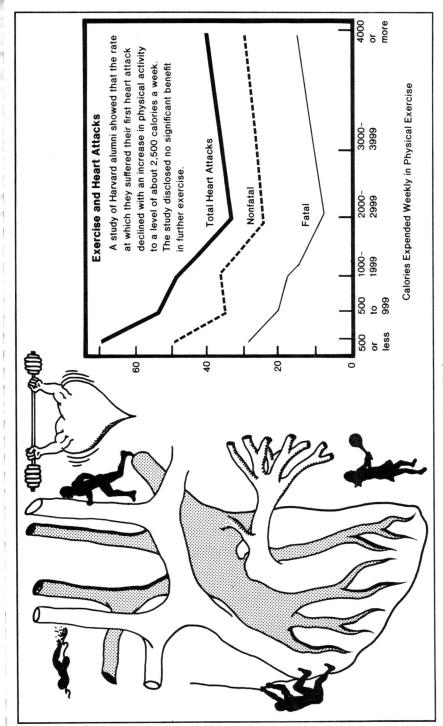

Exercise and Heart Attacks

A study of Harvard alumni showed that the rate at which they suffered their first heart attack declined with an increase in physical activity to a level of about 2,500 calories a week. The study disclosed no significant benefit in further exercise.

Total Heart Attacks

Nonfatal

Fatal

Calories Expended Weekly in Physical Exercise

500 or less | 500 to 999 | 1000–1999 | 2000–2999 | 3000–3999 | 4000 or more

From Executive Fitness Newsletter, Rodale Press Inc., Emmaus, Pa., Feb. 7, 1981 issue.

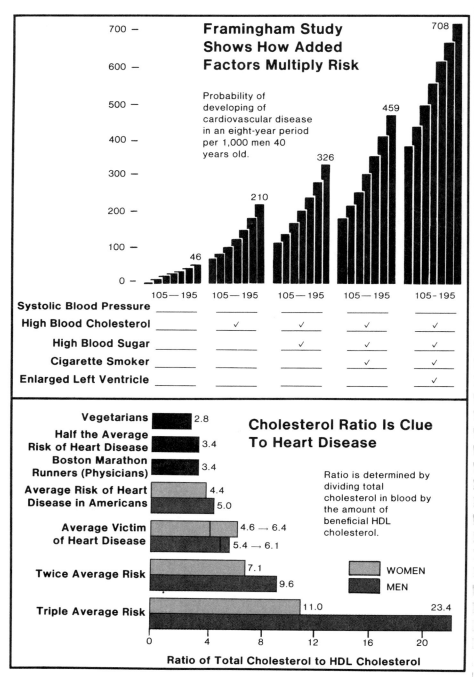

Framingham Study Shows How Added Factors Multiply Risk

Probability of developing of cardiovascular disease in an eight-year period per 1,000 men 40 years old.

Systolic Blood Pressure					
	105—195	105—195	105—195	105—195	105-195
High Blood Cholesterol		✓	✓	✓	✓
High Blood Sugar			✓	✓	✓
Cigarette Smoker				✓	✓
Enlarged Left Ventricle					✓

Cholesterol Ratio Is Clue To Heart Disease

Ratio is determined by dividing total cholesterol in blood by the amount of beneficial HDL cholesterol.

Vegetarians — 2.8

Half the Average Risk of Heart Disease — 3.4

Boston Marathon Runners (Physicians) — 3.4

Average Risk of Heart Disease in Americans — 4.4 / 5.0

Average Victim of Heart Disease — 4.6 → 6.4 / 5.4 → 6.1

Twice Average Risk — 7.1 / 9.6

Triple Average Risk — 11.0 / 23.4

WOMEN
MEN

Ratio of Total Cholesterol to HDL Cholesterol

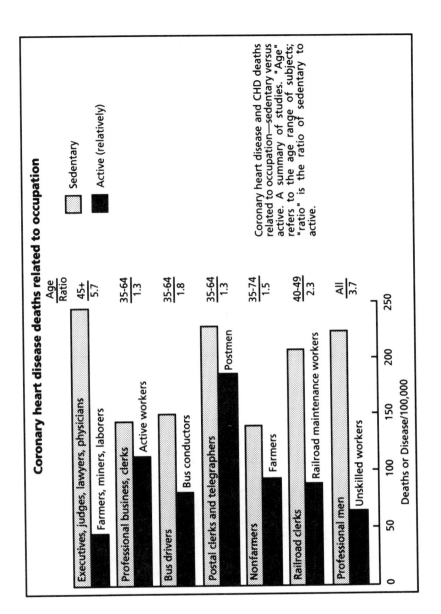

Coronary heart disease deaths related to occupation

◻ Sedentary

■ Active (relatively)

Age	Ratio
45+	5.7
35-64	1.3
35-64	1.8
35-64	1.3
35-74	1.5
40-49	2.3
All	3.7

Executives, judges, lawyers, physicians
Farmers, miners, laborers
Professional business, clerks
Active workers
Bus drivers
Bus conductors
Postal clerks and telegraphers
Postmen
Nonfarmers
Farmers
Railroad clerks
Railroad maintenance workers
Professional men
Unskilled workers

Deaths or Disease/100,000

Coronary heart disease and CHD deaths related to occupation—sedentary versus active. A summary of studies. "Age" refers to the age range of subjects; "ratio" is the ratio of sedentary to active.

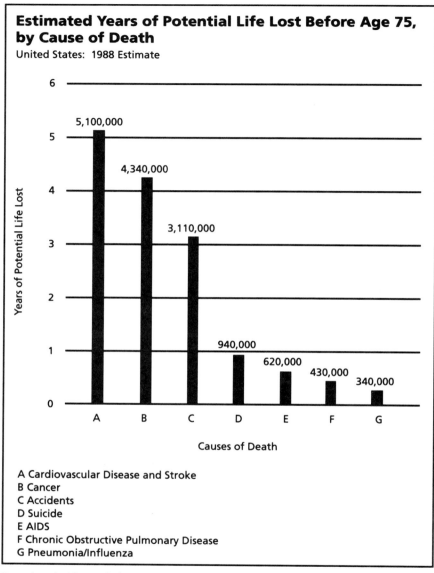

Estimated Years of Potential Life Lost Before Age 75, by Cause of Death

United States: 1988 Estimate

A Cardiovascular Disease and Stroke
B Cancer
C Accidents
D Suicide
E AIDS
F Chronic Obstructive Pulmonary Disease
G Pneumonia/Influenza

Reproduced with permission. From *1992 Heart and Stroke Facts,* 1991. Copyright © American Heart Association.

The study conducted by Dr. Ralph S. Paffenberger Jr. of Stanford University indicates that those men who use more than 2,000 calories a week in exercise had death rates one-quarter to one-third lower than the least active people even if the exercisers were not active prior to graduation.

The study further showed that exercise could diminish potential health threats posed by cigarette smoking and high blood pressure. Expenditures of 2,000 calories a week is the equivalent of walking briskly 20 miles a week. Advantages of exercising beyond 3,500 calories a week are minimal and suggest that moderate exercising may provide as much benefit as very strenuous exercise. As Dr. Paffenberger states "There are lots of skeptics who say people are active because they are healthy. I believe you're healthy because you're active."[7]

Symptoms of Heart Disease

Many people fail to recognize the symptoms (signs) of cardiovascular defects. Often these symptoms are generalized and may indicate a number of problems. The symptoms may be mild or severe but they should be checked promptly in any event.

The symptoms of heart attack are:

▶ shortness of breath

▶ pain in the chest running down the left arm

▶ dizziness, lightheadedness

▶ swelling in the extremities

▶ headache

▶ fatigue

▶ vague indigestion

Summary

Heart disease is the leading killer in the United States. Heart disease is striking more people in their 20s and 30s than ever before. The risk of heart disease depends on several factors. Some factors cannot be controlled by you; these include age, sex, and heredity. Older people, men, and people with family histories of heart disease seem to be more susceptible to heart disease. The controllable factors that contribute to heart disease are elevated blood lipids or fats (cholesterol and triglycerides), elevated blood pressure, obesity, smoking (length of time and amount of cigarettes per day), and lack of exercise. You should recognize the symptoms of heart disease. They include shortness of breath, pain in the chest running down the left arm, dizziness, lightheadedness, swelling in ankles, headache, fatigue, and vague indigestion.

No matter what a person's age, moderate exercise not only improves all-around health but also appears to ward off early death.

▶ Regular exercisers have lower mortality rate and morbidity from cardiovascular disease than do sedentary people.

▶ Research has supported the fact that light-to-moderate exercise is better than remaining inactive. Inactivity carries with it a risk almost as high as the relative risk of smoking a pack of cigarettes a day.

▶ Exercise effectively reduces or prevents the effects of most risk factors such as high blood pressure, obesity, blood lipid profiles, and cigarette smoking.

▶ Exercise after a myocardial infarction may decrease mortality.

Exercise will:

1. Increase coronary collateral circulation.

2. Reduce blood lipids (fats) and change its composition (HDL & LDL).

3. Control body fat.

4. Control high blood pressure.

5. Increase tolerance to stress.

(To evaluate heart attack risk level, see Laboratory 7.)

Exercise: The CHD Prescription

In 1989 a report prepared by a United States Preventive Services Task Force recommended that physicians advise all patients to engage in regular physical activity. In the last 25 years more than 40 major scientific studies have linked exercise to cardiovascular health—morbidity and mortality. Though a number of controversies remain, there is general agreement that exercise exerts a positive impact on many health variables.

Exercise scientists regard aerobic capacity as the best indicator of fitness level, since it represents the functional capacity of the cardiovascular system. In addition, it is accepted as a measure of the health status of the heart, blood vessels, and lungs.

Exercise is a valuable tool in modifying those factors that put people at risk of CHD. People who exercise are less likely to smoke than those who are sedentary. Also, with regard to every level of smoking (from not at all to heavy), exercisers have a lower risk of developing CHD. Other predictors of CHD such as obesity, blood pressure, blood lipids, family history, and blood glucose levels are all affected favorably by exercise.

Apparently, study results indicate that not a very large increase in activity and fitness is required to reduce the risk of CHD. Exercise should be undertaken with consideration given to the following components:

▶ Aerobic activities that involve large muscle movements will promote cardiorespiratory improvement. (See chapter 6.)

▶ Muscular strength and endurance exercise can supplement aerobic exercise and aid in enhancing health and fitness as well. (See chapter 6.)

▶ Exercise should occur three to five times per week and last from 20 to 60 minutes each time.

▶ When fitness improves, a decision must be made regarding continued change or maintaining the achieved level, that is, creating a change or preventing a change from occurring.

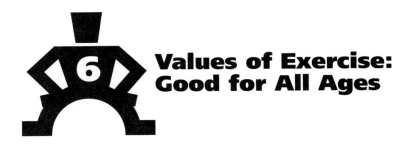

Values of Exercise: Good for All Ages

Preventative Values—Cause of Death

"If exercise could be packed into a pill, it would be the most widely prescribed medicine in the nation."

—Joseph N. Butler, M.D.,
National Institute on Aging

The annual vital statistics report released by the U.S. Department of Health, Education, and Welfare indicates that disease of the heart represents 38.4% of all deaths each year in the United States. Cerebrovascular disease (strokes) kill another 10.9% and arteriosclerosis an additional 1.7%.

These diseases, as previously noted, are most critical to individuals who have defective or weakened cardiovascular systems. The cardiovascular system of an individual cannot always be aided by exercise. Certainly a hereditary defect cannot often be cured, and scar tissue damage to the heart cannot be reversed. In fact, exercise may be ill-advised for people whose cardiovascular systems have limited capacity to respond to exercise stresses. Exercise, however, can have a distinct positive effect upon the variables that make a person vulnerable to cardiovascular weakness.

Cholesterol and blood lipids have been reduced in the blood of people who exercise vigorously. The exercise must be continued on a regular basis to maintain the lowered cholesterol level. The rise in plasma triglyceride level after high-fat meals is considered less in exercised people than resting persons.[8] Long-term exercise programs have been noted to reduce the general level of blood lipids in combination with diet. A diet low in fat produces a sharp reduction in the atherosclerotic effect (heart attacks and strokes) whenever the diet was reduced in fat intake and limited in caloric intake. The combination of diet and exercise is the key factor in the reduction of atherosclerosis.

High blood pressure is easier to control than to cure. We do not fully understand the role of heredity, chemical composition of the body, stress, and lack of exercise in the elevation of blood pressure. Exercise has been found to lower postexercise blood pressure and people who exercise on a regular basis have a better chance to maintain normal blood pressure. It is thought that exercise relieves emotional stress, which can elevate blood pressure, and helps to build a larger cross section of blood vessels so that there is less resistance to the flow of blood through the arteries.

Obesity is a significant contributor to early death through cardiovascular disease. Unfortunately, "there is evidence that during each decade after age 25 the body loses about 3% of the metabolically active cells. If this loss of tissue is replaced, it is probably replaced by fat tissue."[9] The change in our metabolic rate and our choice of high-calorie foods will also contribute to an overfat condition.

Body weight is maintained through a combination of sound diet and exercise. We probably could not lose or maintain body weight without both essentials. Exercise can be a significant part of the control. Overfat youngsters are generally found to eat in a similar manner to their peers but lead sedentary life-styles. A change of exercise pattern that enables you to burn off several additional calories could forestall creeping obesity.

Exercise at All Ages

We are beginning to understand that exercise is important to people at all ages and not to the young alone. There is good reason to believe that proper physical activity can significantly delay the aging process and that regular, proper exercise can help a person to adjust to any stressor throughout his or her lifetime.

As we age, our psychological thoughts and physical needs change slowly, but consistently. As youngsters, thought centers on toys and treats. As teenagers our attention turns to fashions and females or males. Between ages 20 and 40 we concentrate on career and family. Then, "40-something," which brings with it concern for health and longevity.

Americans spend some $2 billion a year trying to counter the effects of aging and tens of billions more trying to disguise aging—hair color, face-lifts, and other cosmetic surgery techniques. These can do little to counteract our natural internal biological aging.

Research is supporting the knowledge that the true "fountain of youth" can be found in our genes and can be enhanced by our life-style choices—exercise and diet in particular.

The childhood years are a time in which the individual approaches the maximum in motor skill and physiological function. Sedentary youngsters are already beginning the process of atherosclerosis that continues into adult life. Autopsies done on American servicemen during the Korean and Vietnamese wars indicated a general condition of atherosclerosis that could be minimized by exercise. Exercise is also needed to preclude adult onset obesity as higher energy expenditure will balance caloric intake. The opportunity for exercise is usually afforded during the preadolescent and adolescent periods as job responsibilities are minimal. The advent of television has provided another choice of sedentary activity that curtails physical activity. Research by Dr. Jean Meyer and other researchers has found that moderate exercise tends to slightly suppress hunger and this is an important contributor to weight control.

It is estimated that as many as 25% of children in the U.S. are obese. The prevalence of obesity among children 6 to 11 years old increased by 54% between 1963 and 1980. Increased physical activity decreases childhood obesity, particularly when accompanied by nutrition education. In addition to reducing or controlling body fatness, exercise will enhance lean body mass and bone structure, which are vital for growing children.

Research has supported the contention that prolonged television viewing is a health hazard to children, according to an American Academy of Pediatrics position statement. TV viewing averages 3 to 3½ hours per day and that does not include games or video recordings.

The habits gained during the childhood years are important precursors for the future. Vigorous, continuous exercise should be part of the habit formation.

Adulthood is often a period of self-imposed inactivity. The stress of occupations as well as the changing manner in which people use their recreational time tends to minimize the amount of vigorous physical activity in which to participate. The change of activity level and the use of high-calorie foods often leads to inevitable creeping obesity, which adds to the risk of heart attack.

Any activity that is part of a person's physical activity as a child can be continued into adulthood. Dr. Peter Wood and members of the Stanford Heart Disease Prevention Program studied 41 middle-aged men who ran at least 15 miles a week and a control group of nonrunners. They concluded that the blood lipid level of the runners was considerably lower than the nonrunners and placed them in a low risk category for heart attack. Similar studies, particularly with marathon runners, who perform best at ages 25 to 35, indicate that people are capable of performing strenuous work throughout middle age.

The senior years can be a time of continuing exercise in a rational manner. Modification of activity may be dictated but exercise programs can improve seniors' physical condition. Herbert DeVries, in work sponsored by the U.S. Department of Health, Education, and Welfare, conducted a study with 41 people aged 50 to 87. He found a 4.9% drop in body fat, 6% reduction in diastolic blood pressure, and a 9.2% rise in maximum oxygen consumption among people in a controlled jogging situation. The number of older people who participate in vigorous training programs is certainly increasing and evidence indicates that exercise is helpful in minimizing the aging process.

An autopsy performed on Clarence DeMar, a cancer victim who ran his last marathon at 69, indicated that his coronary arteries were at least twice as large as normal. Larger coronary arteries are helpful in preventing heart attack and the amount of oxygen made available to the body through this superior delivery system should play a part in mental alertness regardless of your age. You can continue to exercise throughout your adult life and you will feel better for it.

Dr. Thomas Stephens (1988) analyzed four health surveys for evidence that physical activity affects mental health. In a report for the National Center for Health Statistics he concluded that if mental health is defined as including positive mood, general well-being, and relatively infrequent symptoms of anxiety and depression, then physical activity is positively associated with it. One of the Canadian surveys reviewed by Cooper analyzed women's "happiness" scores in relation to their total energy expenditure (activity). With energy output beig equal, "happiness" scores were higher when women engaged in purely recreational activities than when recreation and housework were both part of the activity combination.

The activity a person chooses should obviously be one that is enjoyable and done within the limits of the physical environment and the accessibility of the exercise area. Again, care should be taken that the exercise program is proper for the physical condition of the participant.

Dr. Lester Breslow and his colleagues showed a 520-percent difference in death rate between those who followed seven simple health practices and those who didn't. It should be no surprise that one of the principle health habits is physical exercise.

One of the most common conditions of older people, particularly women, is **osteoporosis.** This disease is a gradual loss of calcium from bones, causing them to become brittle and prone to fracture. Osteoporosis is a result of insufficient calcium intake coupled with lowered levels of sex hormones—estrogen and testosterone. In addition, new information has led medical science to appreciate the importance of exercise in the prevention of the osteoporotic process.

Muscle tissue tends to atrophy as age increases. This is analogous to having a limb in a cast for a prolonged period of time, as inactivity causes a decrease in size of muscle fibers. The rate at which this occurs is slower in fit individuals when compared to unfit. Regular weight-bearing and/or resistance exercise aids in maintaining muscle tissue size and strength at acceptable levels. Recent research has indicated that strength training undertaken by individuals in their 60s, 70s and 80s can produce tremendous gains in muscular strength.

Function deteriorates as bodies age. This deterioration can be slowed if adequate fitness levels are maintained. Exercise should not be viewed as a panacea, but rather as an important part of a healthy life-style.

If a list were to be compiled indicating the changes commonly identified with the aging process and another list indicating the deteriorations induced by forced inactivity, the two would be virtually identical. It would appear that the search for a "fountain of youth" be continued on foot—rapidly.

More than 5,000 Americans turn 65 each day. Many have continued to achieve excellent athletic performance after 55 years of age in such activities as Masters Track, Senior Tennis, and Senior Golf. Perhaps the most impressive performer was Larry Lewis, who ran the 100 yd dash in 18.6 seconds at *102* years of age. Our aging population has more time for leisure and travel at all economic levels. We must have the stamina to enjoy this leisure time. To this end, many fitness programs that are worthwhile endeavors have been developed for older citizens.

Projected Life Expectancy

Age Now	Life Expectancy in years	
	men	*women*
25	76.2	83.1
45	77.3	82.8
65	80.6	84.9
85	90.5	91.9

Office of the Actuary, Social Security Administration
"Life expectancy increases with age, therefore to live to a ripe old age, stay alive as long as you can."

Physical Exercise and Stress

The pace of modern-day life may literally be killing us. This statement is a simplification of the theories developed by several noted individuals. Those in the medical profession include Drs. Meyer Friedman, Ray Rosenman, Hans Selye, and Thomas Holmes.

Dr. Hans Selye is the leader in the study of stress and its effect on the human body. He defines stress very simply as *"wear and tear on the body."* His studies have led to the formation of the **General Adaptation Syndrome** (GAS), which depicts the reaction by the body to a stress (real or imagined). The GAS has three phases: the **alarm stage,** which involves the immediate biochemical changes preparing you to deal with the stress; the **resistance stage,** which involves a "fight or flight" situation; and the **exhaustion stage,** which represents the inability to adjust to stress.

Stress may be regarded as anything that causes change in the body. There are psychological/emotional stresses that raise blood pressure, increase heart rate, create tension in muscle, and alter the chemical balance of the body. The responses are called **psychosomatic,** that is, the mind changing the body.

Exercise is also a form of stress, since it changes physical function in the body, that is, heart rate, blood pressure, chemicals, and muscle tension. These responses are short-lived, occurring during the exercise, and in the long run produce positive changes in function called the **training effect.** Exercise seems to relax the body so that the negative effects of psychological stress do not have the impact on function to the extent of creating harm (stage of-exhaustion).

Exercise is important in lessening the damaging effect of emotional stress. Selye believes that disproportionate stress on one organ or system of the body can be equalized by distributing the stress over a wider part of the body through exercise. Keeping the body fit will help it to withstand external stresses, whether emotional or physical. Exercise and its resulting fitness seem to be able to change the mind; thus, a **somatopsychic** chain of events occurs, that is, the body changes the mind.

Regular exercise, which has been referred to as *"nature's best tranquilizer,"* clearly allows you to feel better. Feelings of well-being associated with exercise have been traced in part to naturally occurring hormones called **endorphins** (endogenous morphine). Both physiological and psychological mechanisms are in effect during exercise and it is difficult to distinguish the exact role that endorphins play in creating a "feel good" sensation.

Hippocrates, the Father of Medicine, reportedly used exercise to treat people suffering from depression. The ancient Greek idea was to treat a problem with its opposite. Consequently, for depression and its accompanying lethargy the remedy was activity.

Drs. Friedman and Rosenman believe that personality determines how an individual handles stress and in that light consider stress to be a cause of heart attacks. Their Type A personality displays hostility, aggressiveness, and impatience. Type A personalities seem to be in a hurry in speech patterns as well as action. They cannot relax or put thoughts of the job out of their minds. "In the absence of Type A Behavior Pattern, coronary heart disease almost never occurs before 70 years of age, regardless of the fatty foods eaten, the cigarettes smoked, or the lack of exercise. But when this behavior pattern is present, coronary heart disease can easily erupt in one's thirties or forties."[10] Type B personalities do not suffer from a sense of urgency and are not overly boastful. Their physical recreation is marked by a feeling of fun rather than overassertiveness. They relax easily and work without undue agitation.

The Type A personality has been found to be more vulnerable to heart attack. The effects of the emotional stressor in conjunction with the variables discussed in chapter 5 make the Type A a high-risk candidate.

Some characteristics of Type A personality are:

▶ explosively accentuate words in normal speech

▶ move, walk, eat rapidly

▶ exhibit impatience

▶ try to think or do two things at once (polyphasic thinking)

▶ control conversation to your own interests

▶ feel guilty when relaxing

► have no spare time

► try to do too much in too short a time

► display characteristic gestures or nervous tics

Dr. Thomas Holmes has devised a scale that quantifies stress. By accumulating "stress points" the chance of suffering poor health becomes greater. Holmes's "Social Readjustment Scale" helps to predict potential for physical illness as the result of emotional stressors. The death of a spouse, divorce, and loss of job would be significant contributors to potential ill health. Even vacations bring additional stress (see Laboratory 14 for further consideration).

Physical exercise has traditionally been used to fulfill the need to "blow off steam" or relax through enjoyable physical activity. Thus, physical activity becomes an outlet for the pent-up feelings caused by stress. Dr. Herbert DeVries has found that exercise had a greater calmative effect when compared with the effects of a tranquilizer. DeVries's findings have since been confirmed by research indicating that strenuous exercise produces hormonal changes in the brain that are akin to tranquilizers. Research on runners, in particular, shows a loss of tension and a relaxed state through exercise. This is important, since it is related to both physical and mental well-being. The need to achieve personal satisfaction through physical activity can be a means of achieving positive mental health.

These positive aspects of sound mental health include a feeling of personal satisfaction and increased self-esteem resulting from a sense of accomplishment. A research study done at Purdue University undertaken by Ismail showed that self-confidence increased considerably as a result of a program of regular exercise.

Most adults will choose recreational physical activity in which they succeed. The sense of accomplishment is important to a person's self-esteem since it may be the only sense of satisfaction or gratification if the person does not enjoy success in occupational endeavors.

Noted psychiatrist Karl Menninger places significant emphasis on play (physical recreation) in the therapy programs of mental hospitals and the maintenance of sound mental health.

Menninger says that *play* differs from *work* in four respects:

1. The means rather than the end is the important thing as far as the player's avowed and conscious efforts are concerned.

2. Pleasure in the activity is more regularly conscious.

3. The activity is consciously dissociated from reality.

4. The aggression motives are more obvious.[11]

Thus, physical recreation, properly chosen, provides a high level of satisfaction because it allows the person to play hard in an atmosphere completely removed from the pressures of the job.

Physical exercise *can* provide experiences that are rewarding beyond the important physical changes that take place in the body. Exercise contributes to emotional stability as it provides for constructive release of tension and provides elements of personal satisfaction. The energy released through exercise is important to the stability of the individual.

Dr. Robert Elliot, an international expert on stress and heart disease, suggests the following ways to cope with stress.

1. "Clarify your values. It's important to run not on the fast track, but on your track. Pretend you have only six months to live. Make three lists: the things you have to do, want to do, and neither have to do nor want to do. Then, for the rest of your life, forget everything in the third category.

2. Improve your "self-talks." We all talk to ourselves, and many of our self-talks are needlessly negative. Discipline yourself not to overreact emotionally. Why despair when sadness is sufficient? Why be enraged when simple irritation will get your message across?

3. Learn how to relax. All you need is a quiet room. Get comfortable. Then close your eyes, breathe rhythmically (preferably from your abdomen), and blot out distractions for 10 to 15 minutes. Do this twice a day.

4. Exercise regularly. Try to exercise at least three times a week for 20 minutes at 75 percent of your maximum predicted heart rate. To determine that rate, subtract your age from 225 (if you're 40, for example, the rate is 185; 75 percent of that, 139, would be age 40's exercise rate). Make sure your doctor approves, and start gradually.

5. Get the leisure you need. The best way to avoid burnout is to allow yourself proper leisure to renew your commitment to work and recharge your batteries. If you're a workaholic, consider: you owe it to yourself to take time off or else you jeopardize your chances of keeping on top of a rough job over the long haul.

6. Adopt dietary goals. Maintain normal weight. Limit fat to no more than 30 percent of your calories; substitute cereals and breads for fats and sugars; moderate salt intake. Also, remember to eat a **real** breakfast.

7. Avoid "chemical haze." One definition of stress is loss of control; the need to acquire control through artificial means accounts for the popularity of nicotine, alcohol, caffeine, and drugs. My advice:

▶ Smoking—Don't. Stopping is the single best thing you can do for your health.

▶ Drinking—Only in moderation. No more than two drinks a day—preferably wine or beer with meals.

▶ Coffee—Too much can make you jittery, irritable, prone to headaches.

▶ Drugs—Only if prescribed. Chemicals make you feel you're in control; but you're not. Real control takes effort, not escape."[12]

Summary

Exercise reduces the blood lipids if a person exercises vigorously over a length of time. Exercise has also been found to reduce blood pressure levels and serves a significant role in controlling body weight. Research is beginning to show that exercise is important to people of all ages and that a rational program of exercise can be carried out through adulthood with beneficial results. Exercise is important emotionally as well as physically. Higher levels of physical fitness appear to delay all of the causes of mortality primarily due to lowered rates of cardiovascular disease and cancer.

The National Institute of Mental Health has summarized what is accepted as consensus agreement about the influence of exercise on mental well-being.

▶ Fitness is positively associated with mental health and well-being across all ages and for both sexes.

▶ Exercise is associated with the reduction of stress and the indicators of stress: muscular tension, resting heart rate, and certain hormone levels.

▶ Common symptoms of the failure to cope with stress—mild to moderate anxiety and depression—can be decreased through exercise.

▶ Some psychological problems, for example, severe depression, require professional treatment, and exercise may be used in addition to medical therapies.

Rx for Life Quality and Quantity: Exercise

Can exercise slow down the inevitable changes in biological function that occur as a result of aging? The consensus appears to be, yes, at least to the point where a physically active life-style can positively affect age-related decreases that are attributed to the fact that most people tend to exercise less as they age. The cardiorespiratory system is favorably affected relative to the ability to supply, deliver, and use oxygen, that is, aerobic fitness. This means that an active 60-year-old could be as aerobically fit as a sedentary 30-year-old. The effects on heart rate, blood pressure, stroke volume, blood volume, and blood chemistry account for this fitness response.

Strength training can forestall and apparent musculoskeletal deterioration that accompanies aging. In many studies, individuals who engaged in resistance training programs gain or at least maintain their strength when compared to inactive people. This reverses the typical downward spiral of muscle mass/strength losses and skeletal bone density decreases that usually accompany the inactivity of aging. Activity will reduce and control the accummulation of body fat that usually accompanies reductions in lean body mass (muscle).

Investigation has created a list of changes in the body that are attributed to aging—muscles, bones, cholesterol, blood pressure, psychological factors, oxygen supply and delivery. Interestingly, if you were to compile a list of changes that occur due to inactivity, they would be virtually identical!

Regular exercise can and does slow down many of the debilitating effects of aging. Irrefutable evidence exists to support the idea that practicing sound principles of exercise can make a contribution to improving and sustaining an independent life-style for all your years.

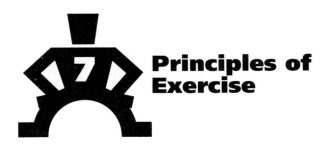

Principles of Exercise

Your body is a remarkably adaptable organism. As such, the systems of which it is composed will adapt to nearly anything. The changes in the body resulting from the physical demands of exercise, as mentioned in previous chapters, are forms of beneficial adaptations. They are positive in nature, thus creating an improvement in potential and function called the training effect. When no physical demands are placed on the body, negative adaptations occur allowing a decline in potential and ability to function—a classic example of "use it or lose it."

Most people will admit that exercise is beneficial. Logical questions to consider would be:

▶ What kind of exercise?

▶ How much exercise?

▶ How often should I exercise?

▶ How hard should I exercise?

There are probably as many kinds of exercises as there are people who are doing them. What is necessary to remember is that in order for the optimal benefit to be gained, exercise must be employed as a "system." *A system of exercise could be defined as planned physical activity performed on a regular basis at a level sufficient enough to induce the training effect.* The training effect is a general term including all the specific positive adaptations created in the body by exercise.

Exercise Variables

In order for the training effect to occur, three variables must be manipulated within the system of exercise. These variables are **frequency, intensity,** and **duration** of exercise.

Frequency—The number of exercise sessions per week

Intensity—The effort level of exercise as measured by heart rate in beats per minute

Duration—The length of time exercise takes place at appropriate intensity levels

When these variables are combined they form an exercise prescription (Ex. Rx.). The use of an exercise prescription ensures that the appropriate exercise variables are combined so that optimal benefits result. The exercise prescription can be designed to produce very specific benefits in the body. For example the Ex. Rx. for strength gain would be different from one for improving cardiorespiratory function.

Frequency—The presently accepted frequency of exercise that is necessary to induce the training effect is three times per week. Although more often is very common and possible, three exercise sessions per week is minimum. These three sessions should be separated so that the body undergoes alternate days of work and recovery.

Intensity—How hard or vigorous must the exercise be to create the training effect? As a general rule the activity must be vigorous enough to raise the heart rate to approximately 120 beats per minute. Individually, a person must exercise at between 60% and 90% of maximum heart rate to assure optimal gains. Intensity is the most critical variable in attempting to create beneficial change in the body. Additional research has indicated that, although a 60% to 90% heart rate level is ideal, lower levels can produce equivalent benefits when combined with adequate frequency and duration. For example, intensity levels at 40% of maximum heart rate are sufficient for some individuals and will allow for a more tolerable effort. As a general rule, when intensity levels are decreased, duration and frequency levels should be increased.

A method of determining an ideal individual target heart rate was developed by Dr. Matti Karvonen. This mathematical formula yields an ideal target heart rate adjusted for age and present resting heart rate level. (See Laboratory 9, Part B for computation procedure.)

Example: If someone were 25 years of age and had a resting heart rate of 80 beats per minute the exercise heart rates at 60% and 40% would appear as follows:

1. Estimated maximum heart rate = 220 minus age
   = 220 − 25
   = 195

2. Estimated maximum heart rate − resting heart rate = adjusted rate: 195 − 80 = 115

3. Work rate = Adjusted rate × 60%; 115 × .60 = 69; Adjusted rate ×
   40% 115 × .40 = 46

4. Training rate = work rate + resting heart rate 69 + 80 = 149; 46 + 80
   = 126

Therefore, a heart rate of 149 represents the exercise heart rate at the 60%
level and a rate of 126 represents the 40% level, a difference of 23 beats per
minute—a very large difference relative to tolerability during exercise. Food
for thought: Research has shown higher intensities create higher dropout rates
from exercise programs.

The chart that follows shows average maximal attainable heart rates for
specific age levels and the respective "target zones." The target zone represents the heart rates that correspond to those necessary to induce the training
effect.

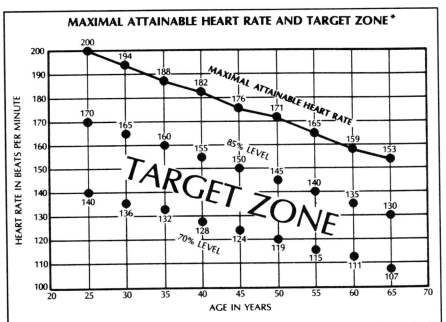

MAXIMAL ATTAINABLE HEART RATE AND TARGET ZONE*

This figure shows that as we grow older, the highest heart rate which can be reached
during all-out effort falls. These numerical values are "average" values for age. Note that
one-third of the population may differ from these values. It is quite possible that a normal
50-year-old man may have a maximum heart rate of 195 or that a 30-year-old man might
have a maximum of only 168. The same limitations apply to the 70 per cent and 85 per
cent of maximum lines.

*Zohman, Lenore, M.D., *Beyond Diet . . . Exercise Your Way to Fitness and Heart Health*, CPC
International, Inc., 1974.

Duration—Once understanding how hard and how often you have to exercise, the next consideration is that of time. Here there is no magic number although general agreement indicates that *15 minutes at target heart rate is a minimum.* The optimal time for best results is between 20–30 minutes of exercise. The length of time here involves the time that the heart is beating at a rate within the target zone.

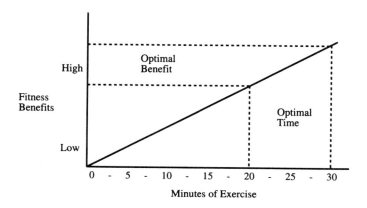

American College of Sports Medicine Recommendations

The American College of Sportsmedicine (ACSM) has developed recommendations on exercise for healthy (asymptomatic) adults. The recommendations include both aerobic and resistance training guidelines, which are summarized as follows:

Frequency—3 to 5 times per week

Intensity—60% to 90% to maximum heart rate; or 50% to 85% of heart rate reserve method using Karvonen determination (see Lab 9) or an RPE rating of 12 to 13 on the Borg scale (see boxed article at end of chapter).

Duration—20 to 30 minutes; or 2½ to 3 miles per workout (if walking, jogging) or the expenditure of approximately 250–300 calories.

Resistance Training—8 to 10 exercises; performed for 8 to 12 repetitions, twice per week as a minimum.

Mode (Type) of Exercise

There are two general types of exercise: *aerobic* and *anaerobic*. Each has specific characteristics related to the biochemistry of energy production in the body. These characteristics are based on the amount of oxygen that can be supplied, delivered, and used during exercise.

Aerobic Characteristics

1. Sustained exercise for 15 minutes or longer

2. Gross (total) body movement (big muscles are active)

3. Repetitive movement (same pattern repeated)

Anaerobic Characteristic

1. Exercise that forces a slowdown or cessation of activity in less than 3 minutes.

The same exercise (running, for example) can be an aerobic effort for some people and anaerobic for others. This is due to individual differences in fitness level that reflect the ability to supply, deliver, and use oxygen. The primary factor in determining whether an exercise is aerobic or anaerobic is the intensity of effort. Generally, high-effort levels are anaerobic and lower-effort levels are aerobic.

How to Exercise

The following chart illustrates a training or *exercising pattern*. It shows the progression from **warm-up,** to **training stimulus level,** to **cool-down.** Please note that exercise at the proper intensity is approximately 20 minutes. The period of time at the 70% to 85% level should be preceded by a warm-up so that the body's systems necessary to support activity are not suddenly taxed. The exercise period should be followed by a gradual return to normal called a cool-down. This allows the body to regain **homeostasis** more easily.

Some of the benefits of a warm-up include:

▶ Gradual increase in heart rate

▶ Gradual increase in blood pressure

▶ Increased blood flow to muscles

▶ Increased muscle temperature

▶ Increased circulatory and respiratory function

The cool-down is an important part of the exercise training pattern. Dilated blood vessels in exercising muscles may cause a fall in blood pressure, pooling of blood in the veins, and diminished return of blood to the heart if exercise is terminated abruptly. When a person walks or engages in other activity involving rhythmic contraction of the leg muscles during the cool-down phase, blood is milked out of these vessels and circulation is aided. The cool-down produces the same benefit as the warm-up, except allowing for gradual decreases in function back toward resting levels.

A proper sequence of an exercise session would be to warm up, stretch, work out, and cool down. Stretching can also be used as part of the cool-down phase.

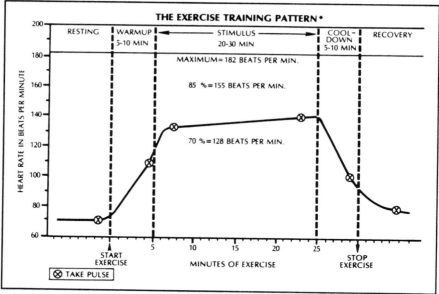

*Zohman, Lenore, M.D., *Beyond Diet . . . Exercise Your Way to Fitness and Heart Health,* CPC International, Inc., 1974.

The Use of S.O.A.P.

In addition to some of the basic considerations of exercise reflecting intensity, duration, and frequency, the idea of S.O.A.P. becomes important. S.O.A.P. not only represents what you should use after exercising, but also the four basic principles related to any exercise program. They are:

▶ **Specificity**

▶ **Overload**

▶ **Adaptation**

▶ **Progression**

Specificity as applied to exercise means that you get what you train for. If your program is strength oriented, the gain will be primarily strength; endurance-oriented activities produce greater endurance. The body adapts specifically to the demands placed on it regulated by the intensity, duration, and types of activities.

To prompt positive change in the body, **overload** must be employed. This principle involves the increase in the demands made upon the body during exercise. Overload can be in the form of greater intensity (strenuousness), duration (longer exercise sessions), or frequency (number of exercise sessions). If resistance training is the type of exercise program, sets, repetitions, and resistance can be forms of overload.

Adaptation is a principle of exercise that merely involves the changes that occur in the body because of the specific exercise program. All aspects of the training effect are examples of this principle.

The last principle of exercise programs is that of **progression.** To induce the training effect in the body you must *progress gradually but continuously.* This principle involves the application of exercise variables that are not too demanding for you but at the same time will be enough to ensure positive gains. On occasion, you may experience **retrogression** in response to any form of overload. During this time your physiology is beginning adaptation, which is manifested in reduced performance level and lingering discomforts. However, this is not a permanent condition, and exercise should be continued at a reduced level after a recovery day.

Maintenance is a principle that should be employed once you are in good condition. It is never necessary to always employ overload. At some point "enough is enough." The guideline is once you look better, feel better, and function better, maintain that exercise prescription; don't overload—anything more is a psychological desire, not a physical need.

Precautions and Considerations

No one exercise program can be used for all people. Fitness goals should be realistic and reflect your needs, interests, and desires—in the present and future. Sometimes, frustration, disappointment, and even a decrease in ability (regression) will occur. It will be helpful in avoiding these possibilities if the following exercise precautions and considerations are kept in mind:

1. Be realistic about what you need and desire from exercise as well as what exercise will and will not do.

2. Choose a form of exercise that will help fulfill your needs, one that will be enjoyable yet demanding.

3. Realize that there are no "shortcut, easy methods" of exercising. It takes time and effort.

4. Choose appropriate clothing for your exercise and the prevailing environmental conditions (temperature, terrain, etc.).

5. Understand that some degree of discomfort seems to be an inescapable adjunct of vigorous muscular activity.

6. If you exercise with someone, try to exercise with a person in the same level of fitness and relative ability and interests.

7. Keep your enthusiasm in perspective; too much exercise— over-stressing—can be dangerous, especially at the start of a program. Some signs and symptoms of *overconditioning* include:

   ▶ Insomnia

   ▶ Prolonged washed out feeling and muscular soreness

   ▶ Extreme weight loss

   ▶ Chronic fatigue

   ▶ Irritability

   ▶ Lowered general resistance (evidenced by sniffles, headaches, fever blisters, etc.)

8. If you are 35 years of age or older, consider it absolutely necessary to have a thorough physical examination before beginning an exercise program. This is especially necessary if you possess any of the heart disease risk factors or have been sedentary for months or years. Even if you are under 35 years of age, a physical exam before starting a program would be an intelligent course of action.

9. Remember, fitness is a lifelong value—to maintain the physical, mental, and emotional benefits, exercise must be a lifetime endeavor. It requires considerable self-discipline, but the rewards are worth the effort.

How much exercise? There does seem to be a point of diminishing return, depending on the person. The following diagram illustrates the fact that beyond a certain point there is little if any benefit. Too much exercise, too often, too hard, and too long is not good.

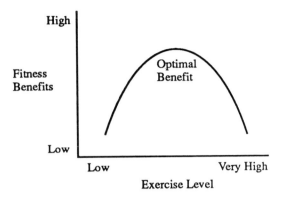

Some Considerations for Exercise and Fitness

▶ The mode of aerobic exercise is not important. Many activities give the same benefit, so choose an activity that you enjoy. Injuries tend to increase with the amount of exercise, so don't overdo.

▶ Low-to-moderate training intensities are best for most adults. Higher intensities increase risk of injury and the probability of becoming an exercise dropout.

▶ Monitor your heart rate on a regular basis when you exercise, on a regular basis but not necessarily every workout.

▶ If your first goal is to lose weight, exercise more often and longer but at low-to-moderate intensity.

▶ Exercising less than twice a week usually does not improve fitness and benefits level off after more than three days per week.

▶ You must keep exercising to preserve your benefit. Cardiorespiratory fitness drops after 10 days of detraining. After 10 weeks you've lost all benefit.

▶ Age does not hinder endurance training. Improvements in fitness in middle-aged and older people can rival those seen in young people.

▶ You need a well-rounded program to exercise all the major muscle groups of the body. Strength training, aerobic exercise, and flexibility exercise are all necessary.

Relative Merits of Various Exercises in Inducing Cardiovascular Fitness*

Energy Range	Activity	Comment
1.5–2.0 Mets** or 2.0–2.5 Cals/min. or 120–150 Cals/hr.	Light housework such as polishing furniture or washing small clothes	Too low in energy level and too intermittent to promote endurance.
	Strolling 1.0 mile/hr.	Not sufficiently strenuous to promote enudrance unless capacity is very low.
2.0–3.0 Mets or 2.5–4.0 Cals/min. or 150–240 Cals/hr.	Level walking at 2.0 miles/hr.	See "strolling."
	Golf, using power cart	Promotes skill and minimal strength in arm muscles but not sufficiently taxing to promote endurance. Also too intermittent.
3.0–4.0 Mets or 4–5 Cals/min. or 240–300 Cals/hr.	Cleaning windows, mopping floors, or vacuuming	Adequate conditioning exercise if carried out continuously for 20–30 minutes.
	Bowling	Too intermittent and not sufficiently taxing to promote endurance.
	Walking at 3.0 miles/hr.	Adequate dynamic exercise if low capacity.
	Cycling at 6 miles/hr.	As above.
	Golf—pulling cart	Useful for conditioning if reach target rate. May include isometrics depending on cart weight.
4.0–5.0 Mets or 5–6 Cals/min. or 300–360 Cals/hr.	Scrubbing floors	Adequate endurance exercise if carried out in at least 2 minute stints.
	Walking 3.5 miles/hr.	Usually good dynamic aerobic exercise.
	Cycling 8 miles/hr.	As above.
	Table tennis, badminton and volleyball	Vigorous continuous play can have endurance benefits but intermittent, easy play only promotes skill.
	Golf—carrying clubs	Promotes endurance if reach and maintain target heart rate, otherwise merely aids strength and skill.

*Zohman, Lenore, M.D., *Beyond Diet . . . Exercise Your Way to Fitness and Heart Health,* CPC International, Inc., 1974.
**Met = multiple of the resting energy requirement; e.g. 2 Mets require twice the resting energy cost, 3 Mets triple, etc.

Relative Merits of Various Exercises in
Inducing Cardiovascular Fitness *Continued*

Energy Range	Activity	Comment
	Tennis—doubles	Not very beneficial unless there is continuous play maintaining target rate—which is unlikely. Will aid skill.
	Many calisthenics and ballet exercises	Will promote endurance if continuous, rhythmic and repetitive. Those requiring isometric effort such as push-ups and sit-ups are probably not beneficial for cardiovascular fitness.
5.0–6.0 Met or 6–7Cals/min. or 360–420 Cals/hr.	Walking 4 miles/hr.	Dynamic, aerobic and of benefit.
	Cycling 10 miles/hr.	As above.
	Ice or roller skating	As above if done continuously.
6.0–7.0 Mets or 7–8 Cals/min. or 420–480 Cals/hr.	Walking 5 miles/hr.	Dynamic, aerobic and beneficial.
	Cycling 11 miles/hr.	Same.
	Singles tennis	Can provide benefit if played 30 minutes or more by skilled player with an attempt to keep moving.
	Water skiing	Total isometrics; very risky for cardiacs, pre-cardiacs (high risk) or deconditioned normals.
7.0–8.0 Mets or 8–10 Cals/min. or 480–600 Cals/hr.	Jogging 5 miles/hr.	Dynamic, aerobic, endurance-building exercise.
	Cycling 12 miles/hr.	As above.
	Downhill skiing	Usually ski runs are too short to significantly promote endurance. Lift may be isometric. Benefits skill predominantly. Combined stress of altitude, cold, and exercise may be too great for some cardiacs.
	Paddleball	Not sufficiently continuous but promotes skill. Competition and hot playing areas may be dangerous to cardiacs.

Relative Merits of Various Exercises in
Inducing Cardiovascular Fitness *Continued*

Energy Range	Activity	Comment
8.0–9.0 Mets or 10–11 Cals/min. or 600–660 Cals/hr.	Running 5.5 miles/hr.	Excellent conditioner.
	Cycling 13 miles/hr.	As above.
	Squash or handball (practice session or warmup)	Usually too intermittent to provide endurance building effect. Promotes skill.
Above 10 Mets or 11 Cals/min. or 660 Cals/hr.	Running 6 miles/hr. = 10 Mets 7 miles/hrs. = 11.5 8 miles/hr. = 13.5	Excellent conditioner.
	Competitive handball or squash	Competitive environment in a hot room is dangerous to anyone not in excellent physical condition. Same as singles tennis.

Note: Energy range will vary depending on skill of exerciser, pattern of rest pauses, environmental temperature, etc. Caloric values depend on body size (more for larger person).
Table provides reasonable "relative strenuousness values" however.
See section on Swimming Programs, p. 28 for information on swimming and cross-country skiing.

Sample Programs: Walking

Distance (miles)	Time (min.:sec.)	Frequency/Week	Points
2.0	24:01–30:00	6	30
3.0	36:01–45:00	4	32
4.0	48:01–60:00	3	33
5.0	60:01–75:00	3	42

Sample Programs: Running

Distance (miles)	Time (min.:sec.)	Frequency/Week	Points
1.0	6:41–8:00	6	30
1.5	10:01–12:00	4	32
2.0	13:21–16:00	3	33
2.0	16:01–20:00	4	36

Summary

The training effect is the change in the body resulting from the physical demands of exercise. Three variables affect the degree of the training effect. They are frequency (how often), intensity (how hard or vigorous), and duration (how long). Among other factors that influence the training effect is specificity. Specificity means that you get what you train for. Another factor is the degree of overload. Overload requires that you place increased demands on your musculature to improve performance. Adaptation is the way in which your body changes as a result of exercise. Progression is needed to continue the improvement of your body's performance until good fitness levels are attained. Then, maintenance of the exercise regimen will help to retain the acquired benefit or training effect.

Listening to Your Body—Perceptions of Work

Exercise intensity (heart rate) is the most difficult variable to deal with in the exercise setting. The ability to exercise at a prescribed heart rate (effort) will vary from person to person even though they may be the same age. Actually, our bodies are usually quite good at letting us know what a "hard workout" is or isn't. The "whole body" perceptions become just as important as a particular heart rate—"my legs are beat," "my lungs are burning," or "this feels easy" are good measures of exertion. This *perceived exertion* is the way in which we can listen to our body and determine sufficient exertion or intensity.

Dr. Gunnar Borg developed a simple method of applying a number value to perceived exertion. It was developed using stress tests (treadmill tests), during which time a patient would indicate how they felt by choosing a number on a scale like the one below.

Very frequently, the perceived exertion will approximate a heart rate. The Rate of Perceived Exertion (RPE) scale is numbered vertically from 6 to 20. A 6 reflects a restful condition with virtually no exertion and a 20 reflects near maximum exertion. The purpose is to combine all feelings—legs, breathing, arms, heart, and so on when choosing one of the numbers. Therefore, it becomes possible to exercise at a particular RPE, based on listening to your body, that coincides nicely with objective measures of exercise intensity like heart rate.

Perceived exertion scale*
6
7 Very very light
8
9 Very light
10
11 Fairly light
12
13 Somewhat hard
14
15 Hard
16
17 Very hard
18
19 Very very hard
20

*The scale was developed in the early 1960s by Swedish physiologist Gunnar Borg. Borg observed that people were quite good at perceiving the physical costs of various work loads. Through several years of research, he constructed a self-report scale to assess these perceptions.

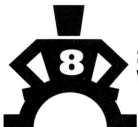

Systems of Exercise— What Do I Do?

If you have asked the question, "What kind of exercise do I do?" a major obstacle has already been overcome. By asking that question you have hopefully admitted (at least to yourself) that exercise is a necessary part of life-style in our society. The answer to the question is . . . "it depends." The type of exercise program "depends" on many factors, such as:

▶ What aspect of fitness do I need most?

▶ What do I want from exercise?

▶ What exercise do I enjoy?

▶ Where will I be exercising (school, home, health club)?

▶ Will I be exercising with someone or alone?

▶ What skills do I need?

▶ Will I need special equipment?

Exercise programs have different outcomes—some will produce gains primarily in endurance; others are conducive to increases in strength, muscular endurance, or flexibility. Some are better for weight gain, others are better for weight loss and a change in body composition. Regardless of what a specific system of exercise will or will not do, all involve a manipulation of the variables mentioned in chapter 7 (frequency, intensity, duration).

Basically, **systems of exercise** can be easily classified into four general categories:

▶ Aerobic

▶ Circuit Training

▶ Resistance Training

▶ Interval Training

Some consideration of each will aid in answering, "What do I do?"

105

Aerobics

Aerobic exercise gained considerable attention primarily due to the professional efforts of Dr. Kenneth H. Cooper, M.D., who is the author of several books dealing with the idea behind aerobics. The term *aerobic* literally means "with air or oxygen." When placed in the context of exercise it includes those exercises which force your body to process large amounts of oxygen without producing or creating an oxygen debt. An inherently aerobic exercise exhibits these three characteristics simultaneously:

1. It can be performed continuously for at least 15 minutes;
2. It involves gross body movement (total body movement); and
3. It involves a repetitive type movement pattern.

The aerobic system of exercise as developed by Dr. Cooper has many distinct advantages: It has adjusted the exercise variables for age, gender, and level of fitness at the start; it has preestablished programs of exercise for various levels of fitness and activity; it tells you how to determine your individual level of fitness (see laboratories pertaining to aerobic fitness); it has established the necessary amounts of exercise to attain and maintain a good fitness level; and the programs have been scientifically formulated based on stringent clinical, laboratory, and field research.

The aerobics system works by using a point system designed to develop cardiovascular efficiency. Exercise performed at a certain activity level will be worth a prescribed number of points based on the amount of energy expended; exercise at a high energy level will earn more points than exercise at a low energy level for the same time period. Points are also earned toward fitness benefit through the duration and frequency of exercise.

According to Dr. Cooper, the exercises that are best for inducing the training effect are running, swimming, and cycling. Points are awarded for many other activities, providing they can be classified as being aerobic.

The aerobics program of Dr. Cooper supports a gradual increase in exercise level until an average of 30 points are being earned on a weekly basis (actual point levels are 27 points for women and 32 points for men). It should be remembered that the primary goal of the aerobics program is to improve fitness levels and thus to impact health status. Consequently, if other goals or needs are desired, this program should be supplemented with other programs. The addition of stretching and strengthening exercises would aid in greater total benefit. The most important factor is to earn the required number of points per week, and not to exercise in a particular manner or at any particular effort level. The following is an example of many exercise programs in Dr. Cooper's book.

Running/Jogging Exercise Program
(Under 30 Years of Age)

Week	Activity	Distance (miles)	Time Goal (min)	Freq/Wk	Points/Wk
1	walk	2.0	32:00	3	13.5
2	walk	3.0	48:00	3	21.7
3	walk/jog	2.0	26:00	4	24.9
4	walk/jog	2.0	24:00	4	28.0
5	jog	2.0	22:00	4	31.6
*6	jog	2.0	20:00	4	36.0
7	jog	2.5	25:00	4	46.0
8	jog	2.5	23:00	4	49.5
9	jog	3.0	30:00	4	56.0
10	jog	3.0	27:00	4	61.3

*By the sixth week, a minimum aerobic fitness level has been reached (36 aerobic points per week), but it is suggested that a higher level of fitness be achieved. By the tenth week of the above program, a total of 61 points per week is being earned, consistent with the excellent category of aerobic fitness. Excerpt from THE AEROBICS WAY by Kenneth H. Cooper. Copyright © 1977 by Kenneth H. Cooper. Used by permission of Bantam Books, a division of Bantam Doubleday Dell Publishing Group, Inc.

Many types of exercise programs are called aerobic. One of the most popular includes **Dance exercise,** also called aerobic dance and jazzercize. All would classify as rhythmically choreographed exercise programs, that is, exercise movements performed to musical background. Most recently, **Step Aerobics** or **Step Training** has come onto the scene. It is a dynamic group exercise program that involves stepping up and down on a platform (varies in height) to music accompaniment. A wide variety of step patterns are included and attempts are made to include upper body strength movements as well.

Circuit Training

One of the most widely used exercise programs is **circuit training.** This method of exercise was developed during the 1950s and is used primarily to improve general body condition. It is truly the "smorgasbord" approach to exercise. Circuit training involves a series of exercises performed one after the other in as continuous fashion as possible. Therefore, since different exercise movements are put together, the end result is some improvement in virtually all aspects of fitness—a smorgasbord effect.

The exercises selected can be of calisthenic type, as is popular in most exercise classes, or involve the use of resistance exercises, which create greater degrees of muscular strength and muscular endurance.

The most common program of circuit training involves 10 to 15 exercise stations or exercises arranged so that they can be performed one after the other. After choosing the amount of work (repetitions of exercise and/or resistance) to be performed at each station, the time to complete three complete circuits is taken. This time is reduced by one-third and becomes a "target time." When someone completes the three complete circuits in the target time, the amount of work at each station is increased (overload principle). A new target time is then established.

The Royal Canadian Air Force developed the XBX (Ten Basic exercises) and the 5BX (Five Basic exercises) programs, which are forms of circuit training.

This form of exercise system can be as simple or as complicated as you care to make it. Exercise movements that involve all major muscle groups should be included.

Resistance Training (Strength Training)

Progressive Resistance Exercise (PRE) is a general exercise system that incorporates three different forms of exercise. This system has been shown to be effective in rehabilitation, increasing athletic performance, and changing physical appearance. The three forms are **weight training, weight lifting,** and **bodybuilding.** All are similar in that they involve the use of resistance (weights) in gradually progressive amounts. However, each is different from the other in terms of outcome of the exercise system. The primary gains for any of the PRE forms are **muscular strength** and **muscular endurance.** The specific gain depends on how the variables associated with this type of exercise system are manipulated. These variables include:

Sets—the number of times an exercise of specific reps will be performed, that is, a group of reps.

Repetitions—the number of times an exercise movement is repeated.

Resistance—the amount of weight that is being moved.

The sets, repetitions, and resistance are combined in an infinite number of ways. Classically, one example of a combination that would guarantee strength gain is as follows:

Sets—3

Repetitions—less than 10

Resistance—10 RM (this would be the amount of weight that could be moved only 10 times, not more—a 10 "repetition maximum")

This combination would change to include the following if muscular endurance and tone were the objective:

Sets—3

Repetitions—15 or more

Resistance—15 RM

Strength training has been studied extensively by many investigators. Differences of opinion based on practical experience as well as the result of scientific research are endless. There is no "one way" to change muscle and its ability to produce force. Recently, one investigator has found that a three set, 6 RM regimen provided the best results when compared to other combinations such as: 5 sets, 8 to 12 RM; 3 sets, 10 to 12 RM; 1 set, 8 to 12 RM. The general rule that can be applied is that increases in resistance ($<$ 10RM) will create strength, whereas increases in repetitions (15RM $+$) will create increases in muscular endurance.

Equipment is necessary in resistance training and may take many forms: barbells, weight plates, dumbbells, Universal machines, Nautilus machines, "heavy hands," and many other types. The cost or sophistication of the equipment do not necessarily determine the end result. The most critical factor in creating muscular strength is the amount of resistance, not its shape. Machines tend to be safer for most people than "free weights" and have been shown to be very productive in aiding muscular change. Machines, free weights, and other devices each have advantages and disadvantages that will affect the individual's choice in selecting one over the other.

Resistance training contributes little if anything to cardiorespiratory fitness, primarily because the actual work phase of exercise is quite short and lasts only a few seconds. Consequently, it does not qualify as an exercise that induces the aerobic training effect.

Weight training is that part of resistance training which involves the use of resistance exercises in the development of strength and/or muscular endurance as an aid in general body conditioning, improvement of sport skills, and changes in body contour (physical appearance) and lean body mass.

Weight lifting involves a competitive approach to resistance training where the primary goal is maximum lift capacity in selected exercises or lifts. Weight lifting is an Olympic sport as well as being an international competitive event. Power lifting is an adjunct form of training and competition.

Bodybuilding practiced by men and women is also a form of resistance training, which has as its goal the creation of maximum muscular hypertrophy and body symmetry. The individuals who enjoy this approach have competition that leads to such IFBB titles as Mr./Ms. America, Mr./Ms. Universe, and Mr./Ms. World. It is not unusual for individuals pursuing this goal to have incredible degrees of muscle hypertrophy. This degree of hypertrophy is not always the normal result of resistance training. Often times anabolic steroids are used to accelerate the growth of muscle and strength. The use of these substances outside of normal medical prescription has significant deleterious effects. Since they alter the normal function of the body, their use should be restricted to medical purposes only.

Relative Adverse Effects of Anabolic Steroids on Males and Females

Liver lesions and cancer	Irreversible clitoral enlargement
Decreased HDL levels	Menstrual abnormalities
Increased serum cholesterol	Aggressive behavior
Increased blood pressure	Psychological disorders
Decreased glucose tolerance	Premature epiphyseal closure in
Testicular atrophy	youths leading to growth
Decreased sperm count	abnormalities
Increased hirsutism (hair	
development)	

Until rather recently, resistance training had been considered the domain of "men only." Fortunately, this taboo has been broken and women have become familiar with the offerings that weight training holds. Contrary to popular opinion the idea of "muscle-boundness" does not occur with this system of training. Women do not have to fear the tremendous degrees of hypertrophy that make them look "too masculine." The reason is that the hormone testosterone will control the degree of hypertrophy and this hormone is present in much higher levels in men than in women. However, there are cases where some women athletes have maximized their inherited tendencies with weight training to produce considerable muscularity.

Isotonic, Isometric, and Isokinetic Exercise

In addition to progressive resistance exercises there are other methods of producing gains in muscular strength and endurance. It must be remembered that changes in muscle tissue can be induced in basically two fashions: **isotonic exercises** and **isometric exercises.**

The difference between the two is that isotonic exercises involve muscular force accompanied by body movement. Isometric exercises involve muscular force with no body movement. For example, a chin-up from a hanging position involves muscular force with the resultant lifting of the body, thus an isotonic exercise. However, if you were to stand in a doorway and "push" out on the door frame, there would be muscular force but no movement, thus isometric.

Isometric exercises will make contributions only to the development of strength and only at the position where the muscular contraction is made (specific portion of the range of motion). It has been advocated that gains in strength can be made with isometric exercises performed once daily for 6 seconds per effort for 5 days per week, providing the muscular contraction is *maximal.* Advantages of isometrics include minimal time involvement, no necessary equipment, and easy-to-understand exercises. Disadvantages include effort at only one portion of the range of motion, the effort *must be maximal* (difficult to measure), and isometrics can become boring. Consequently, motivation is quickly lost. In addition, isometric effort produces a pressure load on the heart that can prove to be detrimental to normal blood pressure responses and should not be used by a person with a cardiovascular problem.

Isometric (static) exercises use less oxygen than isotonic (dynamic) exercises, and isometric exercises often result in a marked increase in blood pressure as the pressure of tensed muscles squeeze blood vessels, limiting circulation. Thus, the heart has to work harder for oxygen. Patients with coronary heart disease should use care with static exercises.

Other derivations of isotonic and isometric exercise include the use of an isokinetic machine. The isokinetic machine is designed to allow for changing resistances (load) as the ability of the muscle to exert maximum force changes throughout a range of motion while the speed of movement is held constant. These machines are used extensively in muscle testing and orthopedic rehabilitation.

Interval Training

One attractive feature of interval training is that *you get to rest.* This rest phase sets this system of exercise apart from others. The idea behind interval training is that greater quantity and quality of exercise can be achieved if the work phase is broken into segments separated by rest phases, that is, more work, less fatigue.

The time of the work segment is alternated with the rest phase, which is also timed. The work phase is usually of short duration because of the high intensity. The rest phase can be either "complete" or "active rest." Complete rest would involve cessation of activity, whereas active rest might include a walk rather than a jog during the rest phase. When a program of interval training is developed for training, it would involve specific "work to rest" time ratios. For example, a ratio of 1 to 3 might mean work 1 minute, rest 3, or rest 3 times as long as the work. By manipulating the work and rest times, "overload" can be controlled. Due to the nature of this combination, cardiorespiratory benefit is the principal gain.

Examples of a part of an interval training system using running as the exercise would be as follows:

1. 10 reps of 100 yards, each in 20 seconds with a 100-yard walk between (approximately 35 seconds).

2. 5 reps of 220 yards, each in 45 seconds, with a 90-second rest between each run.

3. 2 reps of 1 mile, each in 8 minutes with a 5-minute rest between each.

It becomes obvious that by changing the variables the exercise can be made as easy or as demanding as needed.

Previously used only by athletes, particularly track athletes and swimmers, interval training is becoming more popular as a conditioning program adaptable to all people. Many dance exercise classes are including forms of interval training by varying the tempo of music and the effort level of the work.

Cross-Training

Cross-training is a method of combining different exercise types in an attempt to create the elusive "total fitness." This training was originally made popular by the triathlon—swimming, running, and cycling. Traditionally, fitness has been regarded as a measure of aerobic endurance. Cross-training involves developing the five major components of fitness: cardiovascular, muscular strength, muscular endurance, body composition, and flexibility. In a cross-training approach one, two, three, or four "tracks" of exercise can be used. Each track represents a particular form of exercise; for example, combining a swimming workout with two weight-training workouts, with a three-day jogging program.

The advantages to pursuing cross-training may include: overall total fitness; reduction of monotony; enhanced energy expenditure, therefore, fat loss; and reduction of the risk of overtraining and injury.

Step Aerobics

Step Training is the most recent innovation to follow the variety in high-impact and low-impact aerobics. All the rhythmically choreographed exercise programs thrive on variety and this type has captured the current interest. Step training is fairly simple; the choreography is not intimidating, even though some very creative interesting steps and arm movements have been developed; and it can be enjoyed by many exercise enthusiasts. The presence of an instructor (leader), music, and comrades makes it very appealing. Individual fitness levels can be accommodated by using a higher or lower step device.

The systems of exercise thus far considered represent the most popular in use. There are probably as many off-shoots of each one as there are people "doing their own things." Any variation or combination is possible as long as the basic principles of all exercise systems are adhered to: S.O.A.P.

Summary

There are four general classifications of systems of exercise. Aerobics is a system of exercise in which a person will exercise a long period of time before exhaustion. The primary training effect of aerobics is cardiorespiratory fitness. Circuit training uses progressive resistance exercises that have to be completed within a time framework. The desired training effect is muscle strength, muscle endurance, and cardiovascular fitness. Resistance exercises place an overload on a muscle or group of muscles. The overload usually used is a weight or group of weights. The purpose of resistance training is muscular strength and muscular endurance. The principle of progressive resistance exercises can be achieved through isotonic exercises (e.g., push-ups) or isometric exercises (e.g., pushing against a doorway). Each will contribute to muscular strength. Interval training involves maximum effort interspersed with a resting or submaximum phase. The resting time is often shortened as performance improves. The primary result of interval training is cardiorespiratory improvement. For those dedicated to fitness, cross-training is one method of programming that achieves balanced fitness—the elusive total fitness.

Creating a Plan of Action

Exercise can be regarded as a systematic approach to creating or maintaining fitness. Following are some considerations that should help in putting yourself in motion.

▶ Establish realistic goals: Remember, exercise can do great things but there are limitations.

▶ Develop a specific plan: What are you going to do?, how hard?, how long?, how often? Use monthly, weekly, and daily plans.

▶ Involve others for motivation: Seek advice from competent experts (books, videos, personal) and ask others for their support, even exercising with them.

▶ Vary your exercise: Use your plan to establish occasional changes in routine, that is, place, pace, distance, time, sets, reps, resistance, equipment, and so on.

▶ Progress slowly: Life is an endurance effort, not a sprint.

▶ Avoid injury: Be sensible—use good techniques, good equipment, proper warm-up, cool-down, and underdo, don't over do.

▶ Keep a record: Seeing your achievements as a result of your plan provides motivation and information for continued progress.

▶ Reward yourself: Patting yourself on the back to recognize effort and achievement is good to do; tangible results aid motivation.

Examples of Exercise Programs—Recipes for Fitness

To help you select the exercises you need to improve your physical condition or to maintain your present level of fitness it becomes necessary to evaluate the many existent programs of exercise.

It is important to keep in mind several factors that may determine the appeal and consequent benefit attained from any exercise program. Some things to consider in choosing or developing an exercise program are the following:

▶ Present physical fitness levels—reflecting body composition, cardiovascular efficiency, strength, flexibility, and neuromuscular skills.

▶ The need for special equipment or facilities.

▶ Adaptability to a variety of ages.

▶ The specific time requirement for each exercise session.

▶ The relative contribution to the components of fitness.

▶ Adaptability to a variety of locations—school, home, indoors, outdoors, city, suburbs, etc.

In addition to these considerations it must be remembered that if any exercise program is to be of optimal benefit the variables *frequency, intensity,* and *duration* must be employed and adjusted to appropriate age, sex, and fitness levels. By manipulating the variables of exercise it is then possible to create a "cycle" in the exercise program that will aid in avoiding both physical and psychological monotony. This cycle training or "periodization" creates different emphasis on frequency, intensity, and duration as well as type of training during a specified calendar time. For example, approximately every two to four months (eight to sixteen weeks) the emphasis would change to reflect greater frequency, intensity, or duration in the exercise program. Cycling may also include the addition of a different type of exercise into the existing program. For example, resistance training may be added to supplement a jogging program.

You will recall that different exercise programs have different benefits and you must select accordingly. The following examples of programs may help to acquaint you with a variety of possibilities and aid in making an intelligent choice.

Aerobics Program

Dr. Kenneth Cooper developed the exercise system of aerobics based on the relationship between energy expenditure and points. The number of points earned determines the relative fitness level. The best aerobic-type exercises from a fitness standpoint are running, swimming, and cycling. For complete examples of each of these programs as well as others consult *Aerobics, The New Aerobics,* and *Aerobics for Women.* For a starter program see chapter 8, Figure 1.

Following are four examples of aerobic fitness maintenance programs adapted from *The Aerobics Program for Total Well-being* by Dr. Kenneth Cooper. The entire program and their sex and age adjustments can be found in his book.

Sample Maintenance Programs

The following charts illustrate how to maintain 30 or more aerobic points per week.

Included are four programs for walking, running, and swimming; five programs for cycling; and a weekly program incorporating a variety of activities.

Sample Programs: Walking

Distance (miles)	Time (min.:sec.)	Frequency/ Week	Points
2.0	24:01–30:00	6	30
3.0	36:01–45:00	4	32
4.0	48:01–60:00	3	33
5.0	60:01–75:00	3	42

Sample Programs: Running

Distance (miles)	Time (min.:sec.)	Frequency/ Week	Points
1.0	6:41– 8:00	6	30
1.5	10:01–12:00	4	32
2.0	13:21–16:00	3	33
2.0	16:01–20:00	4	36

Sample Programs: Swimming

Distance (yards)	Time (min.:sec.)	Frequency/ Week	Points
300	Less than 5:00	8	30
500	Less than 8:20	5	31
800	13:21–20:00	4	31
1,000	16:41–25:00	3	31

Sample Programs: Cycling

Distance (miles)	Time (min.:sec.)	Frequency/ Week	Points
2.0	6:01– 8:00	20	30
3.0	9:01–12:00	10	30
5.0	15:01–20:00	5	30
10.0	40:01–60:00	4	34
10.0	30:01–40:00	3	40

From *The Aerobics Way* by Kenneth H. Cooper. Copyright © 1977 by Kenneth H. Cooper. Used by permission of Bantam Books, a division of Bantam Doubleday Dell Publishing Group, Inc.

An initial walk-jog-run program may be modeled after the following example:

1st week—3–4 days/week.
  1. Warm-up-stretching and calisthenics 5–10 minutes.
  2. Alternate jogging and walking for 15 minutes.

2nd and 3rd Week—3–4 days/week.
  1. Warm-up-stretching and calisthenics 5–10 minutes.
  2. Jogging and walking for 15–18 minutes.
  3. Run comfortably for 5 minutes.
  4. Walk for 5 minutes.

4th and 5th Week—3–4 days/week.
  1. Warm-up same as above 5 minutes.
  2. Alternate jogging and running for 15 minutes.
  3. Run comfortably for 5–10 minutes.
  4. Walk for 5 minutes.

6th Week—3–4 days/week.
  1. Warm-up same as above.
  2. Jog for 5 minutes.
  3. Run for 15 minutes.
  4. Jog 5 minutes.
  5. Walk 5 minutes.

This progression can be gradually augmented as fitness and tolerance are increased.

An example of a cycling regimen might be as follows:

1. Slow easy cycling as warm-up 5–10 minutes.

2. Harder cycling for 10–15 minutes—heart rate reaching target level.

3. Easy cycling for 5–10 minutes as cool-down.

This kind of general approach may be increased gradually by adding time and increasing speed until one can cycle for up to 30 minutes at 10–15 mph. The approximate caloric expenditure for cycling is as follows:

Approximate Calories Burned Up During Bicyling at Various Speeds

Average Bicycle Speed	55 Lb Person Calories per Hour	110 Lb Person Calories per Hour	165 Lb Person Calories per Hour
5.5 MPH	95	190	285
9.5 MPH	150	300	450
13.1 MPH	235	470	750

Adapted from Raleigh Co. Free Pamphlet, "Bicycling For Fun."

Circuit Training

The term circuit refers to a given number of exercises arranged in a continuous order. It is usually set up in an exercise room or gymnasium and each place where a specific exercise is performed is called a station. The type of circuit is dependent on time, equipment, space, and desired objectives. The Royal Canadian Air Force developed the XBX and 5BX exercise programs, which are examples of circuit training. The 5BX program is composed of six charts involving five basic exercises. These are always performed in the same progression and must be completed in a total of 11 minutes. The exercises include: a flexibility exercise performed for 2 minutes; a sit-up exercise for 1 minute; a back arch exercise for 1 minute; a push-up exercise for 1 minute; and running in place for 6 minutes. As fitness level increases a progression is made from chart to chart until a fitness maintenance level is reached.

The XBX plan for women follows the same general approach except the program involves four charts of 10 exercises. As in the 5BX the starting level on the first chart is based on age and progression and a gradual increase in fitness allowing the work load of each chart to be completed. The Adult Physical Fitness Program based on a circuit training format was a progressive program of calisthenics and endurance activities was developed under the direction of the President's Council on Physical Fitness.

There are exercises for men and women at five levels of difficulty. Progression from level to level is determined by increases in fitness.

The first three levels of the programs for men and women follow and can be found in detail in the book *Adult Physical Fitness* from the President's Council on Physical Fitness in Washington, D.C.

First Three Levels of Adult Physical Fitness Program for Women

Exercise	Level I	Level II	Level III
1. Toe touch	5	10	20
2. Sprinter	8	12	16
3. Sitting stretch	10	15	15
4. Knee push-up	8	12	20
5. Sit-up	5	10	15
6. Leg raise	5 each leg	10 each leg	16 each leg
7. Flutter kick	20	30	40
8. Circulatory activity (choose one for each workout)			
Walking/jogging	1/2 mile (120 steps/min.)	1/2 mile (jog 50 yd.; walk 50 yd.)	3/4 mile (jog 50 yd.; walk 50 yd.)
Rope skipping	2 series (skip 30 sec.; rest 60 sec.)	3 series (skip 30 sec.; rest 60 sec.)	3 series (skip 45 sec.; rest 30 sec.)
Running-in-place	2 min.	3 min.	4 min.

First Three Levels of Adult Physical Fitness Program for Men

Exercise	Level I	Level II	Level III
1. Toe touch	10	20	30
2. Sprinter	12	16	20
3. Sitting stretch	12	18	24
4. Push-up	4	10	20
5. Sit-up	5	20	30
6. Leg raise	12 each	16 each	20 each
7. Flutter kick	30	40	50
8. Circulatory activity (choose one for each workout)			
Walking/jogging	1 mile (120 steps/min.)	1 mile (jog 100 yd.; walk 100 yd.)	1 1/2 miles (jog 200 yd.; walk 100 yd.)
Rope skipping	3 series (skip 30 sec.; rest 30 sec.)	3 series (skip 1 min.; rest 1 min.)	5 series (skip 1 min.; rest 1 min.)
Running-in-place	2 min.	3 min.	4 min.

From the booklet *Adult Physical Fitness,* President's Council on Physical Fitness and Sports, Washington, D.C.

A circuit-training program can be designed in which free weights and/or machines are used. Typically, exercises that involve all major muscle groups are selected and one exercise is performed per muscle group per exercise session. These exercises usually involve multijoint movement and usually 15 to 20 repetitions are performed in only one set. The rest period between exercises is typically very short, usually no more than 15 seconds. The amount of weight or resistance is kept relatively low to allow for the performance of 15 or more repetitions. This type of training can accomplish a great deal in a relatively short workout session.

Weight Training—Resistance Exercise

Care should be taken to select exercises that involve all major muscle groups in the body. This involves a concept called "muscle balance." Muscles function best when all become stronger, and since muscles work in groups, it is prudent to include exercises for all those groups—muscles on the front side (anterior) of the body; the back side (posterior) of the body; the right side and the left side.

Selection of exercises to accomplish this is easy because there are literally hundreds of specific exercises for different muscle groups. The following exercises would fulfill the muscle balance principle with each one having several variations. These exercises can be performed with free weights or with machines such as Universal or Nautilus, among many others.

Squat or Leg Press: for hips, legs, and back

Bench Press: for chest, shoulders, and arms

Military (Shoulder) Press: for upper back, shoulders, and arms

Upright Row: for shoulders and upper back

Bent over Row: for arms, shoulders, and upper back

Curls: for upper arm

Sit-ups or Crunches: for abdominal and trunk muscles

Side Bends: for trunk muscles

The following photographs illustrate these particular exercises.

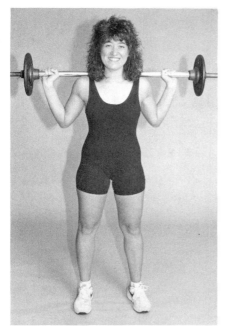 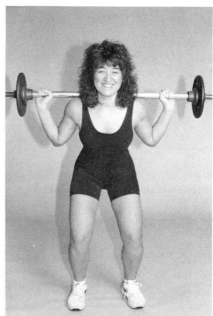

The Squat Exercise: Support weight across shoulders in a standing position; feet are about shoulder-width apart; perform a squat movement until thighs are about parallel to the floor and return to the standing position.

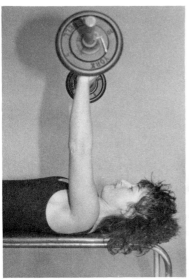 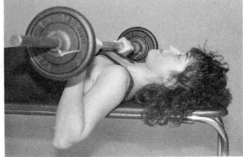

The Bench Press: While lying on a bench, hold the weight with arms straight; then slowly lower until it is contact with the chest; then push up to the starting position with the arms straight.

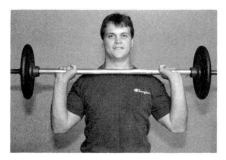
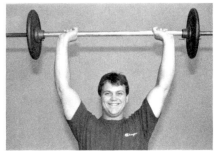

The Military (Shoulder) Press: Begin with the weight supported across the front of the chest with hands about shoulder-width apart; then push the weight up until the elbows are straight and then return to the starting position.

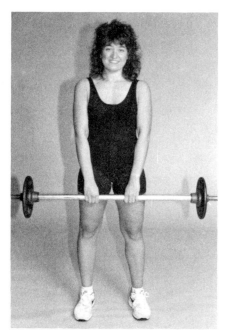
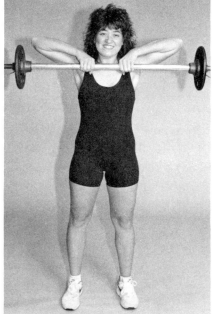

The Upright Row: In a standing position, hold the weight across the thighs with the arms straight; then pull the weight up until the hands are at neck level and return to the starting position.

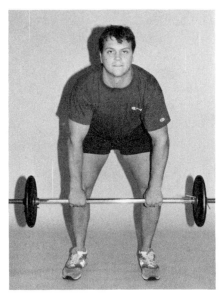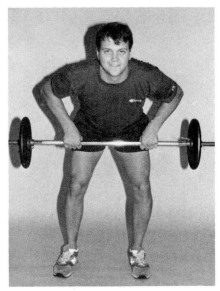

Bent over Row: Begin with the weight held at about knee height, hands about shoulder-width apart, chest held parallel to the floor, head up; lift the weight up toward the chest and return to the starting position, thus creating a rowing motion.

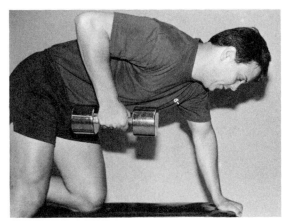

A variation can be performed using a dumbbell and a single arm action with the opposite arm and leg supported on a bench.

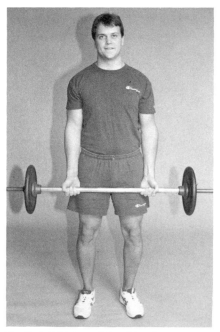 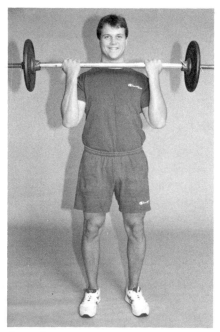

The Curl: Hold the weight with palms up across the front of the thighs with hands about shoulder-width apart. Lift the weight so that the elbows bend and finish with the weight across the body at shoulder level; return to the starting position.

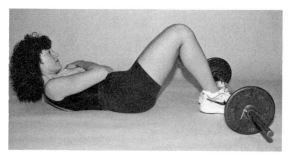

The Sit-up: Start with the toes hooked under a support; hands across the chest; curl the upper body up and then return to the staring position. A twisting motion may be added.

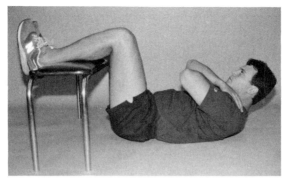

The Crunch: Start with the lower leg on a bench or chair so that the hips and knees are flexed; hands across the chest; curl the upper body up and return to the starting position. This may also be performed with a twisting movement.

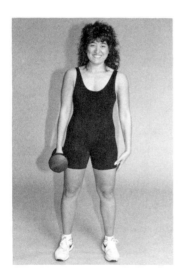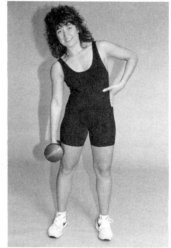

The Side Bend: Start with a weight held in one hand at the side, feet slightly apart; bend to the side and return to the starting position.

Using these exercises while varying sets, reps, and resistances, some basic programs could evolve such as the following:

The "First-Timers" or Starter Program

This can be combined with an aerobic program for enhanced fat loss, lean body mass gain.

Sets—2 to 3

Reps—12 to 15

Resistance—15 RM or about 60% of maximum

Rest—No more than 90 seconds between sets

Frequency—3 days; nonconsecutive

Circuit Set-Up

Sets—1 to 2

Reps—15 to 20

Resistance—20 RM or about 40% of maximum

Rest—less than 15 seconds between sets

Frequency—3 days, nonconsecutive

Basic Strength

Sets—3

Reps—less than 10

Resistance—10 RM or about 70–80% of maximum

Rest—less than 90 seconds between sets

Frequency—3–4 days per week arranged so that 4 days are not consecutive

T and E Program (Tone and Endurance)

Sets—3

Reps—15–20

Resistance—15 RM or about 65% of maximum

Rest—45 seconds to 1 minute

Frequency—3 days; nonconsecutive

Flexibility Exercises—Stretching

Flexibility is the ability of body joints to move through a full range of movement. Bones, muscle, tendons, and ligaments all contribute to this movement. Individuals with good flexibility of joints have greater ease of movement, less stiffness in muscles, and a lesser chance of injury during movement. Exactly how much flexibility you should have is difficult to define. Everyone should try to prevent losses of flexibility that accompany inactivity and aging.

Static stretching (stretch and hold) and ballistic stretching (bouncing movements) are used to create flexibility. The use of fast, bouncing movements can induce the stretch reflex, which can create discomfort and injury. Static stretching is recommended because it does not induce a stretch reflex and is more productive. Any stretching should not progress to the point of pain. Typically, stretching movements should be held for 20 seconds for good benefit.

In some instances more than one stretch held for 20 seconds is advocated and can be performed in sets similar to that of resistance training, that is, three sets of the same stretch can be performed, each held for 20 seconds.

The following figures show some stretching movements that can benefit different muscles and joints of the body.

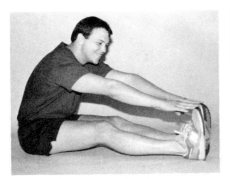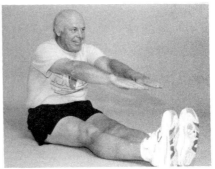

For low back and back of the legs

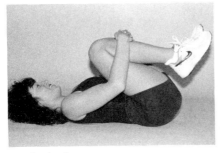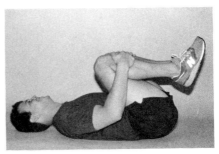

Low back release

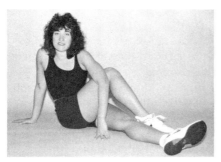
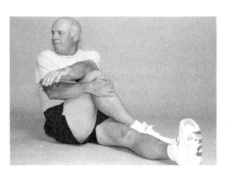

For back, low back, and buttocks

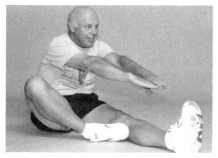
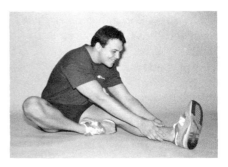

For low back, back of legs, and groin

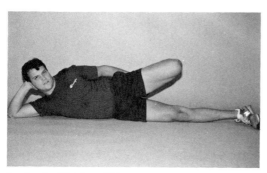

For front of thigh and hip

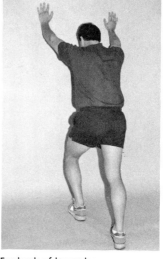

For back of lower leg

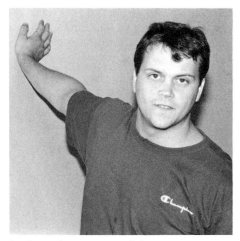

For front of upper arm and chest

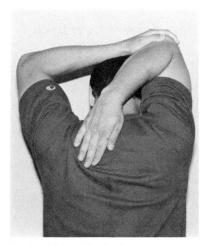

For shoulder and back of upper arm

Interval Training

In recent years interval training systems have evolved for use in competitive athletics as well as general conditioning programs. Interval training stresses the "quality" of work effort as well as the "quantity" found in continuous type programs.

This kind of training involves a higher intensity and consequently should be undertaken after a good base of conditioning has been found.

The following chart shows how to perform an interval training program, using running as an example. In all interval training programs the idea of hard work, brief rest, hard work, brief rest, and so on must be adhered to.

	Distance	Time	Rest	Repetitions
1st Week	220 yds.	40–45 sec.	2 min.	6
2nd Week	220 yds.	35–40 sec.	1 1/2 min.	8
3rd Week	220 yds.	35–40 sec.	1 min.	8
4th Week	220 yds.	35–40 sec.	45 sec.	10
5th Week	220 yds.	35–40 sec.	30 sec.	10
6th Week	220 yds.	35–40 sec.	20 sec.	8

It can be easily seen that as fitness level increases, the amount of rest decreases while the work output remains constant. The variables that may be changed are distance, time, rest, and repetitions.

A similar approach may be used with programs involving walking, cycling, swimming, and weight training, each with its specific benefits.

An Exercise Program for the Low Back

Dr. David Imrie, author of *Goodbye Backache,* has developed a group of simple exercises that build in difficulty to match the ability level of each person's muscles that support the back. The exercises that appear on pages 203–204, correspond to the "tests" that appear in Laboratory 13. Depending on the results, that is, Grade I, II, III, or IV from the measures of this laboratory experience, the appropriate exercise is selected. If results were not good in each of the four measures, then the entire program should be performed at appropriate levels ranging from easy to hard. These exercises can be used to recondition a poorly functioning back as well as to maintain strength and flexibility in a low back that scores well and is pain-free.

Summary

The number of exercise programs are virtually endless. The bases and considerations of selected programs have been presented to aid in developing one of your own. It must be remembered that any program should be based on sound principles of physiology to ensure both safety and benefit.

BACK EXERCISES

	HARD EXERCISES		EASY EXERCISES	
A. **THE** **SIT-UP**	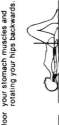 **MAD CAT** Get on all fours and arch your back upwards touching chin to chest. Hold and breathe out deeply.	Now return to the flat position and with your back downwards, like a suspension bridge. Hold and breathe out deeply. 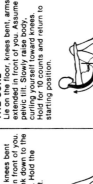	**PELVIC TILT** Lie on your back with knees bent. Place your hand between the "small" of your back and the floor to feel the movement. 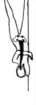	Flatten your back against your hand and the floor by contracting your stomach muscles and rotating your hips backwards. 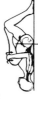
B. **THE** **DOUBLE** **LEG** **RAISE**	**ADVANCED SIT-UP** 1. Sit up with arms folded on chest or 2. Sit up with hands on shoulders. 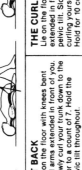	**SIT-UP** Lie on the floor with knees bent and arms extended in front of you. Assume pelvic tilt and slowly sit up keeping feet flat on floor and lower slowly to starting position.	**SIT BACK** Sit on the floor with knees bent and arms extended in front of you. Slowly curl your trunk down to the floor to a count of 7. Hold the pelvic tilt throughout.	**THE CURL** Lie on the floor, knees bent, arms extended in front of you. Assume pelvic tilt. Slowly raise body, curling yourself toward knees. Hold for 10 counts and return to starting position.
C. **THE** **LATERAL** **TRUNK** **LIFT**	**LATERAL LEG LIFT** Lie on your side, one hand under your head and assume the pelvic tilt position. Raise both legs off the floor (2 inches to 6 inches increases difficulty of exercise) and keep body straight. Now raise the upper leg 12 inches, hold and return to starting position. 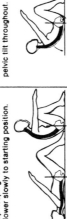		**LEG RAISE** Lie on your side, one hand under your head and assume the pelvic tilt position. Raise upper leg 12 inches, hold and lower.	
D. **THE** **HIP** **FLEXORS**	**PSOAS STRETCH** Lie on back on floor with legs bent. Bend right leg snugly to chest, holding it there with hands. Stretch left leg toward floor. Breathe out slowly as you bend the right leg and straighten the left. Hold for 10 counts. Repeat on other side.		**KNEE TO CHEST** Lie on back with knees bent. Assume the pelvic tilt position. Bend one knee to chest. Use your hands to pull it more snugly to the chest. Slowly return it to starting position. Repeat with other leg.	

From the book *Goodbye Backache* by Dr. David Imrie with Colleen Dimson. Copyright 1983. Used by permission of the publisher, Arco Publishing, a division of Simon & Schuster, New York.

Strolling Through Life

In a competitive sense, walking is a bona fide track event. As a more casual undertaking it can be an incredibly effective strategy for fitness and health.

To begin a walking program, keep in mind that you are in no big hurry—life is an endurance race, not a sprint. For now, forget the watches, heart rates, and distances. Just go for a walk at a comfortable pace somewhere between a stroll and a "hurry-up." You don't have to walk in a particular way but some considerations will help reap benefits.

Posture—Lean slightly forward from the ankles, not the waist. Keep your head level and chin up.

Arm Swing—This makes walking a total body activity. Elbows should be held at a 90-degree angle and arms swing from the shoulder. Hands come up shoulder-high in front and elbows rise on the backswing so that the upper arm is parallel to the ground.

Stride—Make your stride comfortably long and smooth. Remember to step out onto your heel and push off the big toe of the rear foot.

The proper technique is not as important as getting out there and doing something. Schedule regular walks with a friend if you need an extra push; walk first thing in the morning before other commitments creep in; or vary your routine to provide a change in scenery. Maybe you shouldn't think of it as exercise but as time you've set aside for yourself.

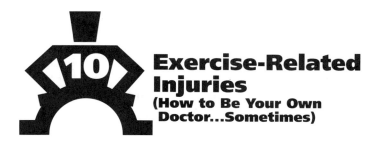

Exercise-Related Injuries
(How to Be Your Own Doctor...Sometimes)

Exercise that is of sufficient frequency, intensity, and duration to produce a beneficial training effect does not go without risk. An inescapable adjunct of physical activity is some degree of discomfort. The discomfort can be manifested in many ways—some injuries are acute (immediate and short term) and others become chronic (long term).

As the exercise population has increased, so has the incidence of related injury. A relatively new area of expertise within the medical profession called *Sportsmedicine* was born of necessity. Sportsmedicine deals with exercise-related injury relative to prevention, diagnosis, and treatment. In 1983–84 the fees for sportsmedicine practice exceeded two billion dollars.

There are many occasions when medical help is necessary and should not be delayed. However, there are other occasions when the recognition, prevention, and treatment of certain injuries can be performed without need for medical assistance. Some common injuries and annoyances warrant consideration so that you might be your own doctor . . . sometimes.

R.I.C.E. as Therapy

The body responds to tissue injury with inflammation (swelling) as it attempts to "cast" the injured part and repair the damage. This inflammatory response causes pain, swelling, redness, and heat. Pain can be reduced, inflammation kept at a minimum, and normal movement resumed if early treatment is begun.

The use of R.I.C.E. in the immediate treatment of injury is a widely advocated procedure in dealing with new injuries. Each letter represents a portion of the treatment to be used.

R = **rest.** Do not continue exercise. Rest may mean 3 days, 3 weeks, or 3 months depending on the injury. In many cases it may involve resting (not using) the injured area not the entire body. For example, a person with a sprained ankle could swim or perform upper body resistance exercise but walking, jogging, or cycling would be out of the question.

I = ice application. The injured area should feel cold to the touch, but be careful not to frostbite. Generally, ice may be applied for 15 minutes and removed for 30 minutes as often as possible for the first two to three days. For chronic injury, ice should be applied after exercise sessions to reduce any inflammation.

C = compression. An ace bandage can be used to hold ice in place as well as to provide compression (gentle squeezing). Compression of the injured area limits the swelling and resulting pain. Numbness, pain, and cramping are signs of too much compression. Always begin compression (wrapping) from a point furthest from the heart, working toward the heart.

E = elevation. Every attempt should be made to keep the injured area at the level of the heart or higher. If the injured part is below the waist, the person should lie down or elevate the part on a stool, chair, or bed while sitting. If the injury is to the arm, wrist or hand the part should be kept at shoulder level with appropriate support.

The R.I.C.E. approach should be continued for at least 48 hours after the injury has occurred.

Remember, to minimize the risk of exercise-related injury:

▶ Underdo exercise rather than overdo

▶ Exercise at your own pace or tolerance

▶ Warm up *and* cool down

▶ Be well-rounded: include flexibility, strength, and endurance in your program

▶ Be progressive; gradually increase exercise level

▶ If it hurts, STOP!!

Types of Injuries

Muscle soreness.   DOMS—delayed onset muscle soreness. This common problem usually appears within the first 12 to 24 hours following exertion. Many theories relate the discomfort to chemical changes in the muscle, fluid accumulation, and microscopic tears in the muscle fiber and connective tissue (the epimysium and perimysium). The soreness may be very significant and persist for one to two days. It will gradually diminish. This discomfort/pain may be relieved by taking aspirin, unless you are sensitive to this substance, in which case an aspirin-free medication containing acetaminophen may be used. In addition, light massage, gentle static stretching, and mild exercise will prove helpful, if tolerable.

Blisters.   A localized problem caused by friction, which creates heat and results in tissue damage and fluid accumulation. Oftentimes "hot spots" can be felt before the actual blistering of the skin occurs. At the site of this friction, fluid begins to accumulate between the layers of skin in an attempt to prevent further tissue damage. This fluid may be clear in color or bloody, creating a "blood blister."

Once a blister has formed it can be extremely debilitating and painful. If the blister has broken, it must be treated as if it were an open wound; that is, it must be cleansed, sterile dressing applied, and it must be kept clean. If the blister is unbroken, two approaches may be considered. First, it may be protected from pressure by applying appropriate gauze padding over the blister or cutting a foam "doughnut"—a circular-shaped piece of foam with a hole, which is slightly larger than the blister size, cut in the center. Second, the blister may be punctured at its side with a sterilized needle to release accumulated fluid. Then it must be treated with an antiseptic and covered tightly. The dressing must be kept clean to reduce the chances of infection. Never remove the layer of skin that covers a blister. The skin covering will aid in protecting the sensitive underlying layer of skin.

Strain.   A tear in a muscle sometimes referred to as a muscle pull. Most times it is caused by an abnormal or excessive muscular contraction. A severe weakness and a loss of function are indications of this condition. Ice applications and compression are recommended for pain reduction and minimization of hemorrhage. Rest and a gradual return to activity are to be expected.

Sprain.   A traumatic injury occurring at a joint resulting in damage to the supportive structures, that is, ligaments. The damage can range from microscopic tears to a complete avulsion (break) of the ligament(s). Immediate application of ice and an elastic compression bandage is advocated accompanied by no weight bearing for as long as 24 to 48 hours, depending on the severity.

Tendinitis.   An inflammation of the specialized fibrous tissue that connects muscle to bone. This condition is created over a period of time and is usually chronic. It should be treated as soon as possible with as many forms of moist heat as are available. Ice application may be used to ease the acute discomfort of an existing condition. Extended rest with activity held to a minimum is advisable.

Contusion.   Results from a hard blow to some part of the body (usually soft tissue). This contact results in a hemorrhage (bleeding) within the tissue involved. There is no break in the skin. The result is pain and tightness in the region of the injury. Immediate application of ice and elastic wrap is necessary to minimize the hemorrhagic tendencies.

Heat Injuries.   Most heat-related problems involve a combination of high environmental temperature, high humidity, and dehydration (less than adequate fluid levels in body tissue). Signs of heat problems include muscle cramps, excessive fatigue, diminished coordination, nausea, and dizziness. All symptoms may appear simultaneously and are classified as **hyperthermia** injuries.

1. **Heat Stroke** is a true medical emergency. This condition may occur suddenly without the classic symptoms. It is characterized by hot, dry skin and a rising body temperature, which may reach 106°. Every attempt must be made to cool the body—ice massage, cool water immersion, and any other means for immediate cooling. Seek medical aid immediately.

2. **Heat Exhaustion** is characterized by profuse sweating accompanied by dizziness and extreme weakness. On occasion unconsciousness may ensue. Fluids should be taken immediately and continuously until symptoms/signs have passed. Physical activity should be halted and attempts should be made to cool the body—cold water, wet towels, ice massage, and shade.

Hypothermia (low body temperature).   Occurs when the heat production of the body is exceeded by heat loss. Symptoms (felt by the involved person) include intense shivering; muscle tensing, fatigue, numbness, drowsiness, and disorientation and stumbling. Hypothermia usually occurs in extended exposure to cold weather and may be accompanied by frostbite. The best approach is to prevent low body temperature from occurring. The most critical concern is the wind chill factor. Layers of clothing that are loose fitting are more effective in conserving heat and thereby preventing hypothermia. See the following chart for the wind chill index and danger zone.

Wind Chill Index									
Actual temperature	With wind blowing at speed, in m.p.h., listed below, it feels as if the temperature is:								
	Calm	5	10	15	20	25	30	35	40
+30	30	27	16	9	4	0	−2	−4	−6
+20	20	16	4	−5	−10	−15	−18	−20	−21
+10	10	6	−9	−18	−25	−29	−33	−35	−37
0	0	−5	−21	−36	−39	−44	−48	−49	−53
−10	−10	−15	−33	−45	−53	−59	−63	−67	−69
−20	−20	−26	−46	−58	−67	−74	−79	−82	−85
DANGER AREA									

Courtesy of THE RECORD.

Summary

There are truly a multitude of exercise-related problems. The medical profession has realized the birth of specializations, which include sport podiatry, sports psychology, and sports gynecology. The chances are great that you may never have any injury-related problem while being involved in an exercise program. In the case of severe injury or prolonged discomfort, it is advisable to seek professional medical evaluation and treatment. Many injuries are "activity-specific," for example, a contusion would be more common in racquetball than in a jogging/running program. By approaching exercise prudently and scientifically, one can minimize any misfortune. Many times the nature, cause, and resultant treatment is very individual, and it is possible to be your own doctor . . . sometimes.

Doing Something Is Better than Doing Nothing—Keep It Going

Injury doesn't necessarily mean a complete breakdown in the exercise routine or exercise itself. Although altering your exercise program to accommodate an injury may be frustrating, good initial care will save days, weeks, and months of potential problems.

Most injury can be viewed as a "temporary inconvenience." The injury may not allow you to do what you always did but total rest is usually not necessary. You can "rest and treat" an injury, yet continue to exercise. An injury may force you to take a break from some form of exercise, but others are available. Someone with an ankle sprain or Achilles tendinitis may not be able to walk, jog, run, or do step training, but circuit training and swimming provide alternatives.

Unfortunately, people tend to resume their old activity schedule too soon when the injury is feeling better but not yet healed. This can be devastating and delay full healing. Remember, you can be your own doctor sometimes, but other times professional advice from physicians, physical therapists, and athletic trainers is the road to travel.

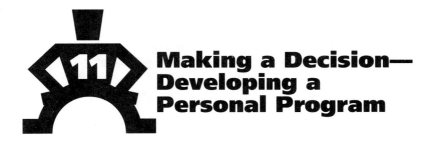

Making a Decision—Developing a Personal Program

Where Am I Now: Determining a Starting Point

An exercise program must start somewhere. It is important to recognize your present level of fitness and begin a program appropriate to that level of fitness.

An initial exercise program that is *too strenuous* can be self-defeating, as it causes muscle soreness, undue fatigue, and a sense of discouragement. A strenuous program can also be dangerous if your physical condition is too poor to adapt to the training.

Generally, a person over 30 years of age should have a thorough physical examination before beginning an exercise program. Certainly, a person of any age who has a physical impairment should check with a physician to determine if a systematic exercise program would cause physical harm.

The starting point for exercise programs is determined by a number of factors, including age, sex, and present level of fitness.

Age. The expectation that youth can do no wrong is enhanced by the fact that the young can initiate exercise programs at any level, adapt quickly, and have little danger of physical harm. As a person matures, the training effect will take longer and, indeed, the eventual goals of the program may be more moderate than for youth. The period of maximum physical maturity is between the ages of 25 and 30. Beyond this point there is a gradual decline in strength and other qualities. Thus, improvement will be slower for a person over 30 and the whole process of reconditioning will take longer than for a younger person.

Sex. Several studies done in recent years indicate that the level of improvement that can be expected by both sexes is generally consistent. Thus, we can expect females to improve performance in the same ratio as males. However, we should not expect the performance level of the sexes to be equal. Women tend to have less muscular strength than males as well as anatomical limitations of speed and endurance.

No one suggests now that equal experience is going to lead to equal performance in all things athletic, or even that the average woman can match the performance of the average man. The physical plant is not the same. Men are bigger and stronger, can run faster, throw and jump farther. But the fact that women are genetically ordained through most of life to compete with less powerful bodies, far from tarnishing their performance, makes it more worthy."[13]

Girls tend to be larger, stronger, and more agile than boys as they approach early adolescence. They can participate successfully in most co-ed activities, including activities, involving strength.

With puberty, the situation abruptly changes. Estrogen levels begin to build in the female body. There is a growth spurt which peaks at about 12 years, then tapers off by 14 or 15. The pelvic bones broaden; breasts and other secondary sexual characteristics appear along with the typically feminine pattern of fat distribution. And menstrual cycles begin. Most boys begin to mature sexually a year and a half to two years later than girls, and then keep on developing much longer, in some cases up to six years longer. As one college athletic director points out, recruiters of women athletes have a singular advantage. "You pretty much know what you are getting, sizewise. While a male athlete can grow a foot or more between freshman and senior year—if you're lucky."

On the average, men end up 10 percent bigger, which happens also to be roughly the increment by which men's Olympic track and swimming times top those of women. However, this gap has been closing so fast over the past quarter-century that there is little reason to suppose it will stop there. Men have longer bones, providing better leverage; wider shoulders—the foundation for a significant advantage in upper-body strength—and bigger hearts and lungs that operate more powerfully and at a slower rate."[14]

The performance level of females has improved remarkably in the last decade because of more intense training and higher levels of female performance. We expect continual improvement in the future.

Present level of fitness.   A critical consideration as to the starting point is the individual's present activity level. An inactive person or a person who is a "weekend athlete" probably has a minimum level of strength, flexibility, and muscular and cardiovascular endurance. (The weekend athlete is the person who attempts to get all his or her exercise in one session a week.) You may determine your starting point by initiating the fitness tests previously described in this text. Most authors of exercise, including Dr. Cooper, describe starting points based on preliminary tests.

Remember: Start slowly.

Work up gradually.

Don't be discouraged.

Underdo rather than overdo.

Individual Goals, Interests, Abilities

The decision about physical activities that are most practical for you depends on a number of factors.

Goals—What do you hope to accomplish? If you are interested in cardio-respiratory endurance you should involve yourself in activities that elevate the pulse rate and maintain the elevation for a considerable period of time before exhaustion. Such activities as jogging, swimming, and bicycling as well as many sports such as soccer, basketball, or field hockey would be appropriate.

Flexibility is achieved by using your muscles and joints through a full range of motion. You must use exercises that actually take you through the complete range of motion. Some sports, such as gymnastics, could also enhance flexibility.

Muscular strength can only be achieved by placing your muscles in overload. Thus, you must work against increasingly greater work loads to achieve your goal.

Muscular endurance is achieved by sustaining an activity for progressively longer periods of time. This goal is usually accomplished by keeping the resistance at submaximum levels and increasing the repetitions of a particular muscle movement.

Skill—How Much and What Kind?

Your chance for success in a sport and your continued participation in that sport will depend on the factors previously mentioned.

Skill is the ability to perform a motor task with ease and efficiency. The components of skill generally consist of *agility, speed, balance, reaction time, power,* and *kinesthetic sense.*

Many people prefer to get their exercise through various sports. They find themselves more easily motivated by sports participation than by a series of exercises and/or jogging. The level of enjoyment in sports may be higher for these people than any other kinds of activity. Sports can contribute to your health if they influence your cardiovascular endurance, muscular endurance, strength, and flexibility.

The skill needed to perform a specific sport may be simple or complex. You may possess the necessary components of skill or you may not. Regardless of the complexity or sport, *most people can learn an activity that will be physically and psychologically beneficial to them.*

Your ability to master a motor skill (sport) will be influenced by other factors as well as your skill components.

Motivation to learn will determine whether you stick to your practice and overcome any difficulties that may appear. Motivation is important because you may become discouraged at slow progress in a complex motor skill such as tennis.

Repetition is important. Motor skills can only be improved through practice. The practice must be sufficient to reinforce the motor skill learned so that you can perform with ease and efficiency. But, remember: *Repetition is only good when you reinforce the right way of doing something.* A golf swing in which the lead arm is not straight will produce inconsistent results at best. Indeed, you may have to unlearn some bad habits gained through incorrect repetition.

Regression is a common factor in the learning of motor skill. Performance levels will periodically diminish or regress. *Don't be discouraged.* You will reach periodic plateaus of performance and then you will continue to improve up to the limits of your ability.

Limitations of Competitive Sports

▶ Seasonal nature

▶ Special equipment needs

▶ Need for teammates or opponents

▶ Amount of time needed for completion

▶ Age will place limits on effectiveness in sports

▶ Does not develop all motor fitness elements equally—each sport stresses only certain elements

Competitive sports can relieve boredom, achieve emotional release, and provide some health-related fitness.

The Criteria for Exercise Training Programs

▶ Require little special equipment or facilities

▶ Can be performed regardless of where you are

▶ Require little time

▶ Need few or no other participants

▶ Adapt to any age or physical condition

▶ Develop health-related aspects of fitness

▶ Exercise all major muscle groups of the body

What Do I Need to Exercise?

Much of the equipment needed for exercise is free. Most of us can run, swim, and do exercises at little cost. Equipment needed to play a sport can be very reasonable or cost several hundred dollars, as in skiing.

What you buy depends on your needs. You may wish to use training devices at home because of your work schedule and the motivation you may derive from their use. It is estimated that Americans spend more than $100,000,000 a year on exercise equipment.

How do you know what equipment is good? Exercise equipment usually requires you to be active or passive on a machine such as an exercycle. Active exercises require you to work while on the machine, often placing your body in an overload situation. Passive exercise enables the machine to work on the individual, as in massaging or shaking the individual. *Passive exercise machines do not work.* They may relax you but they do not build musculature, cause weight loss, or improve cardiorespiratory fitness. Such devices as contour tables, steam cabinets, and belt massagers are of little benefit.

Active exercisers, such as a stationary bicycle, rowing machine, or a weight-training machine, would be of value in an overall exercise program as they may stimulate cardiovascular response or place the muscles in an overload situation. You can buy equipment that is beneficial. But remember, *does it do what it claims to do?*

If the device claims to improve cardiovascular circulation, does it allow the heart rate to increase to 120 and over for a sustained period of time? If the device claims to improve muscular strength, does it allow the exercised muscles to be overloaded enough to create strength gains?

Some devices claim to cause weight loss and/or redistribution of weight. Remember, fat accumulates from overeating and lack of exercise. The only way to reduce the percentage of body fat is to reduce caloric intake and increase exercise.

There is no effortless way to fitness. Your body must work for a reasonable period of time to achieve results. Any program that predicts improvement within less than 15 minutes a day should be suspect.

Home Exercise

Many people are choosing to buy equipment for home utilization. They understand that strength and flexibility training are important adjuncts of cardiorespiratory training and that cardiorespiratory training in climatic extremes (snow, heat) may require indoor exercise. The convenience of working out at home would dictate careful choice of equipment.

The commercial exercise establishments have learned that brightly lighted, airy, attractive exercise areas with shiny, safe equipment are important indicators to exercise. You should attempt to replicate these physical surroundings. Try out equipment in a commercial setting and buy only what you need for your program. Among home equipment possibilities would be treadmills, rowing machines, exercise bikes, multigyms, free exercise weights, cross country skiing devices, and videos.

Treadmills

Treadmills provide the runner with the same benefits that jogging provides and can be used during inclement weather. They also allow you to control your workout by varying the speed at which you run. Running on a treadmill may take some getting used to, but injuries are usually minimal. Aerobic and interval training can be done well on a treadmill.

Rowing Machines

Rowing machines, like treadmills, have the primary benefit of cardiorespiratory endurance and muscular strength benefits, depending on how the machine's resistances are set. The machine can be used as an alternative for a person recovering from a running injury or who has incurred these injuries in the past. Blood pressure tends to elevate, so caution should be used for people with cardiovascular disease.

Exercise Bikes

Exercise bikes also achieve cardiorespiratory benefits in addition to muscular endurance of the large leg muscles. Many chronic knee injuries common to runners can be minimized, and there are some added flexibility benefits to the muscles of the lower back. Use caution initially if you are using the bike as an alternative to running, as you do use some different musculature that could be overextended with initial intensity.

Multigyms

Multigyms provide muscular strength and muscle endurance benefits. They are safe and usually take a minimum of space. The specific equipment you buy will depend on your needs. You can get a circuit-training effect from home gyms, if they are properly equipped. Thus, this equipment can give you all the health-related aspects of fitness with minimal potential for injury.

Free Weights (Barbells, Dumbbells)

Free weights continue to be the best way to achieve muscular strength and muscle tone. The training can be selective and allow you to work with both large and small muscle groups and help achieve a good range of motion with these muscles. Free weights are usually cheaper than multigym systems but the potential for injury from dropping the weights is much greater and they are some times less appealing than multigyms.

We will probably see considerable use of equipment in the home as the costs vary tremendously depending on the complexity and durability of the machines. Health spa memberships of several hundred dollars a year with little utilization might be weighed against similar costs for home equipment that will be used.

Summary

Be sure you are ready for exercise. You can hurt yourself if you attempt to do too much too soon. The exercises or activities you choose will depend on your age, your sex, and your present level of fitness. You should choose an exercise program designed to meet your individual needs. Sports activities require various elements of neuromuscular skill. You should analyze the components of your ability and choose activities to meet your exercise needs and also provide a high level of personal satisfaction. You do not usually need expensive equipment to achieve your goals. Use a bicycle or other piece of equipment if it helps you to achieve your goal. Remember: Get the benefits of exercise while you enjoy yourself. (See Laboratory 15 for evaluation and selection of future activities.)

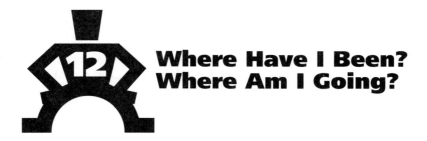

Where Have I Been?
Where Am I Going?

You have reached a point where you must decide how to allocate your recreational time. The particular activity or group of activities you choose should meet criteria that would provide you with meaningful exercise and a sense of satisfaction from your experience. Several factors will affect your selection of activities.

Factors Relating to the Selection of Activities

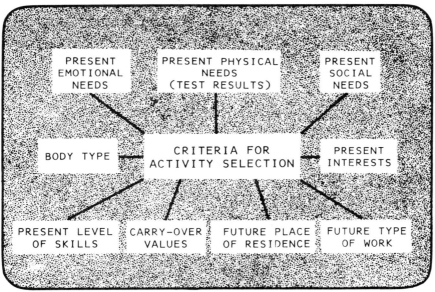

Van Huss, Wayne D. et al., *Physical Activity in Modern Living*, Prentice-Hall, Inc., Englewood Cliffs, N.J., 1969. Reprinted by permission.

Your **present physical needs** will be based on your present level of fitness. Any attempt at beginning an exercise program should be based on what you are capable of doing at the present time. A running, swimming, or other cardiovascular program must be instituted at the proper entry level or you will be discouraged. Programs to improve muscular strength and muscular endurance will also depend on your present physical needs. Remember that inactivity will cause regression and you must start at a lower threshold.

Social needs of people are often satisfied through positive physical recreation experiences. Your interaction with others in sport and recreation will help develop and reaffirm friendships through enjoyable experiences. The communication aspect of physical recreation often allows an opportunity to develop social contacts.

Present interests are, by definition, transitory. Our adolescent interests are marked by an interest in activities that are group oriented (softball, basketball, etc.) as we desire peer recognition, and we are committed to being part of a group relationship. Our interests become more singular as we age, and our desires for personal satisfaction may cause our interests to change. Interests will also be influenced by present popular exercise forms (tennis, jogging) and by the interests of our friends.

Your type of work should influence your choice of activity. A sedentary occupation should be balanced by the choice of vigorous physical activity that contributes to physical and mental well-being. Jobs that entail vigorous physical activity should be complemented by less energetic and more physically relaxing activities.

Future place of residence is very difficult to predict, since we are a rather mobile society and you may be subject to change of geographical area. Climatic conditions do play a part in the intelligent choice of activities. Activities are adapted to the physical and social climate of the geographical location. Warmer climates provide excellent opportunity for outdoor recreation throughout the year (tennis, golf, volleyball). Cold climates provide opportunities for a variety of activities (skiing, platform paddle tennis) and a need to build indoor facilities to satisfy climatic conditions (indoor tennis).

The carryover values of sports and physical recreation activities are critical to your ability to develop lifelong pursuits. Our school years are filled with the need to develop our relationships through group activities. Unfortunately, we often lose interest in these activities as we get older, and we rarely find opportunity to participate in organized recreation including 10 or more people as required in many team activities.

Physical education programs have started to address this problem by introducing dual or individual activities with carryover values. The secondary school programs are often handicapped in offering these programs because of the size of the classes, cost of the program, lack of facilities, and the continued needs of their students, which are satisfied by group activities.

College physical education classes offer an excellent opportunity for you to choose carryover skills. A well-developed college physical education program would enable students to participate in individual and dual activities (tennis, golf, skiing, swimming, backpacking, etc.) as well as activities that improve and provide insight into personal fitness (body conditioning, weight training, and jogging).

Your present skill level will influence your success in an activity. The complex activities will take more time to master. Indeed, you may be limited in your ability to utilize balance, power, speed, agility, reaction time, and kinesthetic sense. Most people can achieve success in a range of physical activities, although they may not achieve an exceptional skill level.

Your body type will be a continued influence on your general body weight as well as your ability to perform activities with ease and efficiency.

Present emotional needs are an important consideration as we recognize the catharsis that physical activity can bring during a troubled day. Articles depicting the emotional release achieved by joggers and long-distance runners have been numerous as have the positive attestments from psychiatrists that physical activity provides a positive release from emotional stress.

Consider all these factors and then embark on a planned program of exercise, for you have learned that exercise can be a dominant force in your lifestyle. The benefits of exercise can measurably improve and sustain the quality and quantity of life.

Exercise can:

▶ Increase heart stroke volume at rest

▶ Decrease resting pulse rate

▶ Decrease exercise pulse rate

▶ Increase recovery rate from exercise

▶ Increase ability to sustain one's self in an activity

▶ Increase the rate at which calories are burned off

▶ Increase muscle tone

▶ Increase muscle strength

▶ Increase muscle endurance

▶ Decrease emotional stress

▶ Increase survival rate from heart attack

▶ Increase recovery rate from heart attack

▶ Increase self-confidence and self-esteem

Exercise, as part of a general life-style that includes proper diet, can contribute immeasurably to your sense of personal worth. Exercise may make you feel better and look better. Try it—just for the health of it!

Filling Time or Killing Time

One phenomenon of our contemporary society is an increase in "discretionary time"—free time, sometimes called leisure time. This discretionary time can be filled or killed—and all too often it is easier to kill time rather than be a participant, easier to be a consumer than a creator, easier to do nothing rather than something.

One approach to using discretionary time is to keep some of it for yourself. Invest time in yourself. Exercise is one such option that allows you to make such an investment. This investment can yield outstanding benefits—physically and psychologically. It may take some looking, some rescheduling, some excluding to find this "self-time," but it can clearly be accomplished. Fill some of this newfound time with exercise—sow an act, reap a habit; sow a habit, reap a life-style.

LABORATORIES

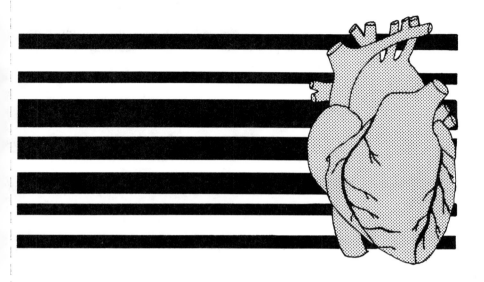

A Thought on Fitness Measurement

The idea of having to submit to some form of physical fitness test generally creates apprehension regarding the age-old "pass or fail" syndrome common to all such procedures. Actually, the fear of "failing" a fitness test is unfounded, because fitness does not come in a "have or have not" package. Everyone has fitness—only the degree of its parts vary. In this sense, what is being done acquaints you with various elements of fitness and how much of these elements you possess as part of your physiology. Hopefully, what will be revealed will encourage you to exercise for the health of it.

▶ Laboratory 1
Exercise Knowledge Tally

Purpose

To critically respond to statements about exercise and therefore gain a better understanding of facts that support or refute the statement.

Procedure

Since this is not a test and no grade is involved, you can be honest in your responses; there is no penalty for guessing. Read each statement carefully and select your response by placing a checkmark or X in the appropriate blank space.

Statement	Definitely False	Probably False	Not Sure	Probably True	Definitely True
1. A lack of exercise as well as no exercise may cause tight shortened muscles	_____	_____	_____	_____	_____
2. All exercise produces the same benefits	_____	_____	_____	_____	_____
3. Regular exercise may help prevent and cure low back pain	_____	_____	_____	_____	_____
4. Regular exercise can make bones stronger	_____	_____	_____	_____	_____
5. For cardiovascular benefit to last, only a single exercise session is necessary	_____	_____	_____	_____	_____
6. Regular exercise tends to raise someone's resting blood pressure	_____	_____	_____	_____	_____

Statement	Definitely False	Probably False	Not Sure	Probably True	Definitely True
7. People who have fit muscular systems also have fit cardiovascular systems	_____	_____	_____	_____	_____
8. Exercise can turn fat into muscle	_____	_____	_____	_____	_____
9. Most problems of excess weight result from hormone problems	_____	_____	_____	_____	_____
10. Static stretching is the best way to improve flexibility	_____	_____	_____	_____	_____
11. Exercising a specific body part or place removes fat from the spot	_____	_____	_____	_____	_____
12. Problems like depression, hypertension, and ulcer may partly be caused by a lack of exercise	_____	_____	_____	_____	_____
13. Walking, running, tennis, and racquetball are all aerobic exercise	_____	_____	_____	_____	_____
14. A regular program need not involve a great deal of time	_____	_____	_____	_____	_____
15. All exercise burns the same number of calories	_____	_____	_____	_____	_____
16. Intensity of exercise is measured by how much you sweat	_____	_____	_____	_____	_____
17. Warm-up has little benefit and should only be performed by those in poor condition	_____	_____	_____	_____	_____

Name _____

Section _____ **Date** _____

Statement	Definitely False	Probably False	Not Sure	Probably True	Definitely True
18. Aerobic exercise must be performed at least three times per week for optimal benefit	_____	_____	____	_____	_____
19. For benefit, target heart rate must be 90% of your maximum	_____	_____	____	_____	_____
20. Calories don't count, only the type of food is important	_____	_____	____	_____	_____
21. Low-calorie diets produce the best weight and fat losses	_____	_____	____	_____	_____
22. Duration, frequency, and intensity are all forms of overload	_____	_____	____	_____	_____
23. Regular exercise can slow down the aging process	_____	_____	____	_____	_____
24. Active people are less likely to have heart attacks	_____	_____	____	_____	_____
25. Research has not shown any relationship of fitness to job performance	_____	_____	____	_____	_____
26. Exercise needs remain the same throughout one's life	_____	_____	____	_____	_____

Statement	Definitely False	Probably False	Not Sure	Probably True	Definitely True
27. The best way to burn fat is to exercise very hard—"no pain, no gain"	_____	_____	_____	_____	_____
28. Using resistance (weight, etc.) is the best way to improve muscle strength	_____	_____	_____	_____	_____
29. Anyone who exercises needs vitamin supplements and extra protein to build muscle	_____	_____	_____	_____	_____
30. If you have an injury you should "work through it"	_____	_____	_____	_____	_____

▶ Laboratory 2
Physical Fitness Appraisal

Purpose

This physical fitness appraisal is designed to objectively assess each student's capacity for specific physiological capacities. The assessment is designed to focus on three important parameters that have been traditionally viewed as strategic in evaluating functional fitness levels. These parameters are cardiovascular efficiency, dynamic strength/endurance, and flexibility.

Part A—Cardiovascular Efficiency—Foster's Test

This test is based on the principle that activity increases heart rate in almost direct proportion to the intensity of the activity. Therefore, if the heart rate increases out of proportion to the intensity, it may be concluded that the subject has low level cardiovascular efficiency. (See Labs 8, 9, and 10 for other methods of determining cardiovascular efficiency.)

Procedure

1. Determine heart rate per minute in a standing position via either carotid or radial pulse (a 10-second count ×6 will suffice). Be accurate since subsequent measures are compared to this heart rate: _____ BPM.

2. Run in place for 15 seconds at the rate of 180 steps per minute (3 steps/second) then IMMEDIATELY take heart rate for 5 seconds (convert to minute rate by multiplying by 12): _____ BPM.

3. Continue standing for 45 seconds and take heart rate again (a 10-second count ×6 will suffice): _____ BPM.

4. With the data obtained consult the following table to determine efficiency rating (a score of 15 points is the maximum obtainable). First, from column A determine the points for your standing heart rate: _____ . Second, find the difference between heart rate after running in place and

the standing rate. Look to column B to determine the respective points for this difference: _____ . Third, find the difference between the heart rate after the 45-second rest and the original standing heart rate.

Look to column C for respective point values: _____ . Fourth, add the point values for the efficiency rating. The higher the rating the more efficient is the cardiovascular system (see example calculation).

Column A points for standing heart rate: _____

Column B points for difference between standing and exercising: _____

Column C points for difference between standing rate and the rate after resting for 45 seconds: _____

    Total points for your cardiovascular rating: _____

A Standing Pulse Rate	Points	B Pulse Rate Immediately Following Exercise Minus Standing Pulse Rate (B − A) Difference	Points	C Pulse Rate After 45-Sec. Rest Minus Standing Pulse Rate (C − A) Difference	Points
100 or less	0				
101–105	−1				
106–110	−2	0–20	15		
111–115	−3	21–30	13	5	−1
116–120	−4	31–40	11	6–10	−2
121–125	−5	41–50	9	11–15	−3
126–130	−6	51–60	7	16–20	−4
131–135	−7	61–70	5	21–25	−5

From Donald Mathews, *Measurement in Physical Education,* Fifth Edition. © 1973 by W. B. Saunders Company. Reprinted with permission.

    Example calculation:

Standing heart rate	= 90/min. (A)	= 0 pts.
Heart rate after exercise	= 120/min. (B − A)	± 13 pts.
Heart rate after 45 sec. rest	= 95/min. (C − A)	= −1 pt.

                        Efficiency rating = 12 pts.

Part B—Strength/Endurance

The following procedures yield a simple assessment for existing muscular efficiency, which focus on specific body areas that, when analyzed, correlate well with the overall muscular system.

Pull-Ups for Men (shoulder girdle and arm strength/endurance)

The subject grasps the bar with the palms facing forward extending the arms and legs fully. The subject then performs as many pull-ups as possible.

A pull-up consists of pulling the body up with the arms until the chin is placed over the bar followed by a return to the extended body position. Partners will stand to the side and count.

Bent Leg Sit-ups for Women (abdominal strength)

The subject lies on her back with the knees bent at approximately a 90-degree angle. The arms should be placed across the chest. A partner holds the subject's ankles and keeps the feet in contact with the floor at all times. Perform as many sit-ups as possible in one (1) minute.

The partner will keep count. A sit-up will consist of raising up from the lying position so that at least the upper half of the back is off the floor or mat and then return to the original position.

Part C—Flexibility

Static Hip Flexion For Men and Women

The subject sits on the floor with the knees together and legs extended. The feet are held flat against a bench inclined on its side. While the partner holds the legs in place the subject reaches forward with both arms fully extended. The degree of hip flexibility is measured by the distance in inches + or − from the toes.

Scoring Norms

Part A—Cardiovascular Efficiency

Approximate Rating

Raw Score	Rating
12–15	Very Good
9–11	Good
6–8	Fair
3–5	Poor
<–3	Very Poor

Part B—Strength/Endurance

Pull-Ups for Men

Raw Score	Rating
15–>	Very Good
11–14	Good
7–10	Fair
4–6	Poor
<–4	Very Poor

Bent Leg Sit-Ups for Women
(1 minute limit)

Raw Score	Rating
30–>	Very Good
25–29	Good
20–24	Fair
15–19	Poor
<–14	Very Poor

Part C—Flexibility

Static Hip Flexion Measure (inches)

Raw Score	Rating
−2–>	Poor
0–−2	Fair
0(touch toes)–+2	Acceptable
+2–+4	Good
>4	Very Good

Name _____

Section _____ **Date** _____

Laboratory 2 Results Sheet

Part A—Cardiovascular Efficiency—Foster's Test

1. Efficiency Rating Score _____

Part B—Strength/Endurance

1. Pull-ups for Men: Number _____ Rating _____
2. Sit-ups for Women: Number _____ Rating _____

Part C—Flexibility

1. Hip Flexion: Number of inches _____

   Rating _____

Based on the results of these measures, which types of exercises and/or exercise programs should be undertaken to improve these three areas of fitness and why? (See chapters dealing with principles and programs of exercise.)

Cardiovascular efficiency:

Strength/Endurance:

Flexibility:

▶ Laboratory 3
Somatotype and Body Composition

Purpose

To explore the interrelationships of body type, metabolism, and weight control so that students can make judgments concerning their own weight-control problems, if any.

Procedure

Place all results on sheet provided at end of this laboratory.

Part A—Subjective Evaluation of Body Type

Researchers have determined that body type is a function of body weight. These same researchers have also identified three basic body types. These are endomorphic, mesomorphic, and ectomorphic. In the extremes, the endomorph is characterized by a soft, rounded body possessing large amounts of adipose tissue, particularly in the abdominal region, the mesomorph by a highly solid muscular physique, and the ectomorph by a slender, delicate physique. Although most individuals fall somewhere between classifications, somatotyping can serve a useful purpose in helping individuals determine a desirable body weight for their body type.

Using the somatotype continuum scale below, rate your own somatotype based on Sheldon's system (see chapter 3). Circle the number you believe expresses the degree of endomorphy, mesomorphy, and ectomorphy, remembering that a low number indicates very little of those characteristics while a high number indicates a great deal. It might be interesting to have a friend give a rating of your somatotype for comparison. Record your estimates on the results sheet.

Somatotype Continuum			
Raters:			
Self	1 2 3 4 5 6 7 Endomorph	1 2 3 4 5 6 7 Mesomorph	1 2 3 4 5 6 7 Ectomorph
Classmate	1 2 3 4 5 6 7 Endomorph	1 2 3 4 5 6 7 Mesomorph	1 2 3 4 5 6 7 Ectomorph

Sample Rating. John Doe might receive a **2** in endomorphic characteristics, a **3** in mesomorphic characteristics and a **1** in ectomorphic characteristics which means his body type, though having some endomorphic characteristics, is more clearly mesomorphic or meso-endomorphic.

Part B—Determining a Desirable Weight

Table 1 indicates a range of weights based on a variance in body type for the heights listed.

Table 1
Desirable Weights for Adults

Height (inches)	Weight (lb)	
	Men	Women
60		109 + or − 9
62		115 + or − 9
64	133 + or − 11	122 + or − 10
66	142 + or − 12	129 + or − 10
68	151 + or − 14	136 + or − 10
70	159 + or − 14	144 + or − 11
72	167 + or − 15	152 + or − 12
74	175 + or − 15	
76	183 + or − 15	

*Heights and weights are determined without shoes or clothing.
*Source: Food and Nutritional Board, National Research Council.

Determine if your weight is appropriate when compared to accepted standards.

1. List your height: _____ in.

2. List your weight: _____ lb.

3. My allowable weight range for height and body type from Table 1:

   from _____ lb to _____ lb.

Name _____

Section _____ **Date** _____

4. I am within this allowable weight range: _____

I am above this allowable weight range: _____

I am below this allowable weight range: _____

Part C—Body Fat Level: Ponderal Index

The above exercise might be sufficient to assess your desirable body weight, but it does not identify your degree of obesity, since obesity does not correlate exactly with being overweight.

To assess one's percentage of body fat a simplified procedure involves a mathematical formula designed to yield a "ponderal index." The ponderal index is a ratio of height to weight. This is calculated by dividing your height in inches by the cube root of your weight in pounds. The accuracy of the method varies, since it comes closest with individuals of average bone structure and proportions. It is least accurate for extremes in body build. This method will, however, yield a "ball park" estimate of body composition.

A chart of cube roots for various weights is indicated below (divide the appropriate one into your height in inches).

91 lbs. = 4.5	149 lbs. = 5.3	226 lbs. = 6.1
97 lbs. = 4.6	157 lbs. = 5.4	238 lbs. = 6.2
104 lbs. = 4.7	166 lbs. = 5.5	250 lbs. = 6.3
111 lbs. = 4.8	175 lbs. = 5.6	262 lbs. = 6.4
118 lbs. = 4.9	185 lbs. = 5.7	274 lbs. = 6.5
125 lbs. = 5.0	195 lbs. = 5.8	287 lbs. = 6.6
133 lbs. = 5.1	205 lbs. = 5.9	300 lbs. = 6.7
141 lbs. = 5.2	216 lbs. = 6.0	

Once you have calculated your ponderal index, find it on the vertical axis of the following graph.

Next draw a line from your ponderal index so that it intersects with the diagonal line on the graph.

From this point of intersection draw a line down so that it intersects with the horizontal axis labeled percent body fat. This will be an approximation of the percentage of your total body weight that is fat.

The example shown on the graph is with a ponderal index of 13 and a resultant percent body fat of 14.

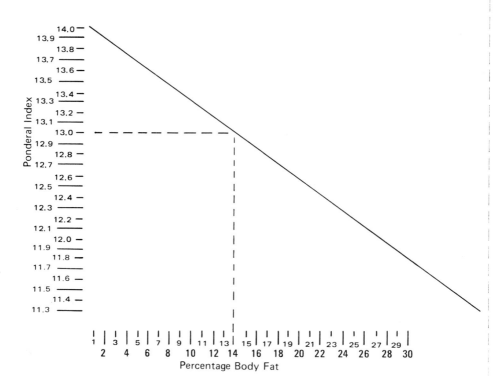

Part D—Determination of Body Composition Via Skinfold Measurement

As explained in the related chapter on body composition, it is not unusual for an individual to fall within the normal range for body weight but actually have excess body fat.

To arrive at an accurate estimate of percent body fat, various skinfold measurement must be taken. To do this, skinfold calipers are used. These measure skinfold thickness in millimeters. Skinfold thicknesses will be measured using the following procedure:

1. The calipers should be held in the right hand with the thumb on the "trigger," which controls the pincers.

2. A skinfold is pinched up at the appropriate site with the thumb and index finger of the left hand. The skinfold should be pinched up along the natural line of the body; for example, with the triceps skinfold, the natural line would produce a vertical skinfold. (All skinfolds taken on dominate side.)

3. After the skinfold has been pinched up, open the pincers of the caliper and place them approximately one centimeter (1 cm) below the thumb and index finger. Let the pincers close on the fold slowly, completely releasing the trigger.

4. After the trigger has been released, count two seconds before reading the meter. This is done because the tissue will compress to some degree.

5. Read the meter to the nearest millimeter and record the findings.

The sites of skinfold measurement: Men take 4; Women take 2.

For Men and Women

1. **The Triceps** (back of the arm): arms at your side; your partner will grasp a skinfold on the back of the arm halfway between the shoulder and elbow. It will be a vertical skinfold. (See appropriate picture.)

2. **The Suprailiac** (hip): halfway between the lower rib and the hip bone (about an inch above the hip) the skinfold should be taken so that it runs horizontally (parallel to the beltline). (See appropriate picture.)

3. **The Subscapular** (base of shoulder blade): along the lower edge of the shoulder blade at a slight angle. (See appropriate picture.)

4. **The Biceps** (front of upper arm): at the point of greatest curvature of the muscle, measured vertically. (See appropriate picture.)

167

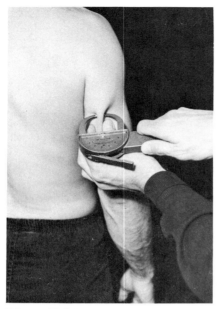

Triceps skinfold

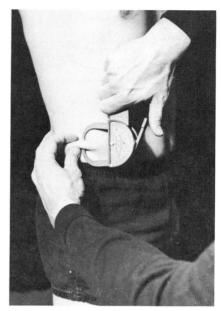

Suprailiac skinfold

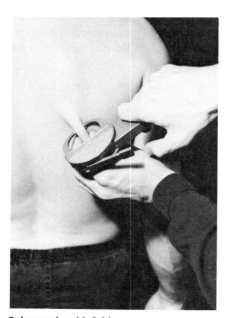

Subscapular skinfold

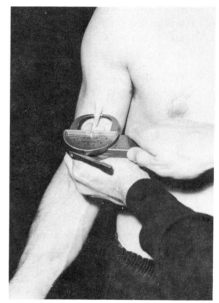

Biceps skinfold

168

Name _____

Section _____ Date _____

Table 2

Women		Men	
Total mm Skinfold	% Fat	Total mm Skinfold	% Fat
8	13	15	5
12	14	20	9
14	15	25	11
18	16	30	13
20	17	35	15
24	18	40	17
26	19	45	18
30	20	50	20
32	21	55	21
34	22	60	22
38	23	65	23
40	24	70	24
42	25	75	25
44	26	80	26
48	27	90	27
50	28	100	28
52	29	110	29
56	30	120	30
58	31	130	31
62	32	140	32
64	33	150	33
68	34	160	34
70	35	175	35
76	37	190	36
80	38	205	37
82	39	220	38
86	40	235	39
88	41	255	40
90	42	275	41
		295	42

From *Activetics,* by Charles T. Kuntzleman. Copyright © 1975 by Charles T. Kuntzleman. Reprinted by permission of the author.

Laboratory 3 Results Sheet

Part A—Somatotype

1. My Somatotype is: _____ — _____ — _____

2. Body type is called a (an): _____

Part B—Skinfold Results

1. Women: Triceps Skinfold _____ mm

   Suprailiac Skinfold _____ mm

   Total _____ mm

2. Men: Triceps Skinfold _____ mm

   Suprailiac Skinfold _____ mm

   Biceps Skinfold _____ mm

   Subscapular Skinfold _____ mm

   Total _____ mm

3. Percent Fat (see table 2) _____ %

4. Weight of Fat in Pounds

   _____ $\times$ _____ = _____
   TBW   **% FAT**   **FW**
                                              (pounds of fat in body)

5. Weight of Lean Body Mass (**LBM**): _____

   _____ — _____ = _____
   TBW   **FW**   **LBM** (in pounds)

6. Determining optimal body weight (this mathematical adjustment will be most reliable if the percent fat exceeds recommended values, i.e., 30% for women; 20% for men.

Optimal body weight = your lean body mass divided by the difference between 100% and the percent fat you would like to be (example: 100% − 15% = 85% or .85)

a. Subtract the percent fat you would like to be from 100%:

100%(1.00) − _____%(.   ) = _____%(.   )

b. Divide the result into your Lean Body Mass (LBM) determined in number 5.

_____   _____

c. The result is your optimal body weight, which is _____ lb.

7. Required **fat** loss = Present TBW − Optimal body weight

Required **fat** loss = _____ − _____

Required **fat** loss = _____ pounds

► Laboratory 4
Ideal Body Weight

Purpose

To mathematically determine your ideal body weight, if such a thing actually exists.

Many attempts have been made to create a method for determining an ideal body weight for men and women. Most are based on the assumption that a perfect ratio of height and weight exists, allowing a predetermined number of pounds of weight for each inch in height.

The greatest fallacy in these methods revolves around the theory that all women and all men have the same somatotypes at all ages. In other words, all women who are of the same height also look alike, so, therefore, they should weigh the same. The identical situation is assumed for men. This is obviously an erroneous assumption.

Procedure

Follow the mathematical process for men and women, respectively, to determine an ideal body weight for your height.

Part A

Men: Standard assumption: 5 feet tall and 106 pounds allowing 6 pounds for each inch over 5 feet tall.

a. 5 ft. = | 106 pounds |

b. Number of inches   = [   ]
   over 5 ft.

$$\times \quad 6$$

[   ]   Number of
              pounds allowed

173

c. Add

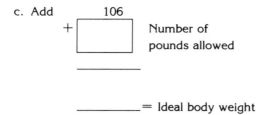

$$+\ \boxed{}\quad \text{Number of pounds allowed}$$

_____ = Ideal body weight

Part B

Women: Standard assumption: 5 feet tall and 100 pounds allowing 5 pounds for each inch over 5 feet tall.

a. 5 ft. = | 100 pounds |

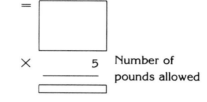

b. Number of inches over 5 ft. = [   ]

×   5   Number of pounds allowed

c. Add

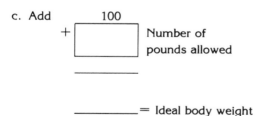

$$+\ \boxed{}\quad \text{Number of pounds allowed}$$

_____ = Ideal body weight

Questions

Is the weight you calculated realistic? _____
Why?

Why not?

174

▶ Laboratory 5
Determining Energy Requirements

Purpose

To assess the daily caloric requirements for basal metabolic requirements and daily activity requirements.

Energy (caloric) requirements vary among individuals, depending on body size, gender, and daily activities. Energy needs are for two main purposes: interval function for life called basal metabolism, and for daily activities. To estimate how much energy (total calories) you need each day, the following **calorie calculator*** is used.

Simply follow the directions to determine the number of calories needed for (1) basal metabolism and (2) daily caloric requirement. It must be remembered that this daily requirement is that needed to maintain present body weight.

Procedure

1. Using a pin as a marker, locate your actual weight on line 1.

2. Setting the edge of a ruler against the pin, swing the other end to your height on line 6.

3. Remove the pin and place it at the point where the ruler crosses line 2.

4. Keeping the edge of the ruler firmly against the pin on line 2, swing the right-hand edge to your sex and age on line 7, using the age of your nearest birthday for the purpose.

5. Remove the pin and place it where the ruler crosses line 3. This gives you the calories used daily (in 24 hrs.) if you are resting and fasting (basal metabolism).

6. To the basal calories thus determined, add the percentage above fasting and resting for your type of activity using the Activity Level Guide. Leaving the pin in line 3, swing the edge of the ruler to the right to the proper percentage on line 5. Where the ruler crosses line 4, you will find the number of calories necessary to maintain your present weight.

*Hewitt, Donald W., M.D., *Reduce and Be Happy*, The Pacific Press Publishing Assoc., Calif., 1955. Reprinted by permission.

Hewitt, Donald W., M. D., *Reduce and Be Happy*, The Pacific Press Publishing Association, California, 1955. Reprinted by permission.

Activity Level Guide for Use with Calorie Calculator

The following percentages should be added depending on daily activities.

20 percent should be added to the basal caloric needs of individuals who are bed patients, or those whose activities are confined to sitting in a wheel chair.

30 percent should be added for ambulatory patients who are in need of more rest than are normal individuals, but who are able to engage in limited physical exercise such as is obtained by short walks.

40 percent should be added for individuals of somewhat greater activity, but whose energy output is still considerably below par. In this class may be cited such persons as housewives who engage in various social activities, but who hire others to do housework and students who are not participating in regular physical activity but are primarily engaged in study. Usually they are nonworking students whose physical activity is primarily limited to walking to and from classes.

50 percent should be added for individuals engaged in clerical duties, various machine operators, cooks, domestics of various sorts, chauffeurs, and others doing similar semisedentary work. Students who work at clerical jobs such as the library or as laboratory assistants are included in this area. Their physical activity includes about two hours of walking or standing daily.

60 percent should be added for manual laborers, truck drivers, farmers of various types, roofers, and the like. Teenager children who are overweight are included in this classification. College students who, in addition to their academic studies, participate in limited physical exercises such as are offered in the physical education activity courses, or intramural sports of a moderate nature are included, as are those students who attend dances and other social activities regularly and walk or stand about two hours each day.

70 percent should be added for individuals who engage in heavy work, such as construction work, mining, and stevedoring. In this group also are college students participating in physical education classes and individual sport and exercise activity programs on a regular, daily basis, and those on intercollegiate teams of a moderate nature with daily practices and weekly contests.

80–100 percent should be added for those engaged in the heaviest type of work described in the 70 percent category, and for those students participating in intercollegiate sport activities that have the highest rate of calories expenditure as shown on the activity chart (basketball, track, etc.).

Laboratory 5 Results Sheet

1. According to the Calorie Calculator, how many calories are being consumed per day, enabling you to maintain present body weight?

   _____ Total Calories

2. Approximately how many of the total calories are used for basal metabolism?

   _____ Calories for BMR

3. Approximately how many calories are being used for daily activities above basal metabolism?

   _____ — _____ = _____
   (total calories)   (BMR calories)   (Activity calories)

▶ Laboratory 6

Calorie Expenditure— Calorie Ingestion

Part A

The amount of energy you burn off during a day depends on your activity. Sedentary activity burns off relatively few calories while activities that use your whole body in strenuous exercise burn off high levels of energy.

Listed below are several activities and the calorie burn-off that occurs during an *hour* of each activity for people of various weights.

1. Record your physical activity for a 24-hour period and place the breakdown of hours in the appropriate space under "No. of Hours."

2. Refer to the chart for calorie value of activities for 1 hour. Multiply the calories expended in an hour for your weight times the hours in activity and record under "No. of Calories."

3. Add up total calories for 24-hour period and record under "Total Calories."

Activity	No. of Hours	No. of Calories
Sleeping		
Sitting		
Walking		
Light—clerical or sales work of equivalent		

Activity	No. of Hours	No. of Calories
Low intensity—housekeeping, bowling		
Moderate intensity—singles tennis, racquetball, walking 4–5 mph		
High intensity—running 6 mph or more		
Sports activities—soccer, football, etc.		
Other recreational activities—tennis, basketball		

TOTAL CALORIES _____

You will note that the energy expenditure for the 200-lb person is twice the expenditure for the 100-lb person doing the same activity. You will also note that vigorous activities do, indeed, burn many calories. Not all activities are listed, but you should be able to make a reasonable determination of energy used in other activities by these examples.

Activity	Calories/Hr. Based on Body Weight				
	100	110	120	130	140
Sleeping	43	47	52	56	60
Lying awake	50	55	60	65	70
Sitting, not working	65	72	78	85	91
Sitting, reading	69	76	83	90	97
Standing, relaxing	69	76	83	90	97
Dressing	77	85	92	100	108
Typing rapidly	91	100	109	118	129
Light exercise, i.e. filing in office	110	121	132	143	154
Walking slowly	130	143	156	169	182
Carpentry	156	172	187	203	218
Active exercise, i.e. volleyball	188	207	226	244	263
Walking average rate	195	215	234	254	273
Severe exercise, i.e. sit ups, push ups	292	321	350	380	408
Swimming, non-competitive	325	358	390	423	455
Jogging	370	407	444	481	518
Very severe exercise, i.e. wrestling, hard running; hard rowing	390	429	468	507	548

Calories/Hr. Based on Body Weight

150	160	170	180	190	200	lb
65	69	73	77	82	86	
75	80	85	90	95	100	
98	104	111	117	124	130	
104	110	117	124	132	138	
104	110	117	124	132	138	
116	123	131	139	146	154	
137	146	155	164	173	182	
165	176	187	193	209	220	
195	208	221	234	247	260	
234	250	265	281	296	312	
282	301	320	338	357	376	
293	312	332	351	371	390	
438	467	496	526	555	584	
488	520	553	585	618	650	
555	592	629	666	703	740	
585	624	663	712	741	780	

Part B

Maintenance of body weight requires an equal expenditure of energy and intake of calories through food. There is a general list of calorie value in chapter 3. Other calories values are available in most cookbooks.

List the calorie values for the food that you have eaten during the same 24-hour period recorded in Part A.

Breakfast		Lunch		Dinner		Other	
Food	Cal.	Food	Cal.	Food	Cal.	Food	Cal.
_____	_____	_____	_____	_____	_____	_____	_____
_____	_____	_____	_____	_____	_____	_____	_____
_____	_____	_____	_____	_____	_____	_____	_____
_____	_____	_____	_____	_____	_____	_____	_____
_____	_____	_____	_____	_____	_____	_____	_____
_____	_____	_____	_____	_____	_____	_____	_____
_____	_____	_____	_____	_____	_____	_____	_____
_____	_____	_____	_____	_____	_____	_____	_____
_____	_____	_____	_____	_____	_____	_____	_____
Total _____		Total _____		Total _____		Total _____	

Total calories for 24-hour period _____

Calorie intake and expenditure vary with each day, so Part A and Part B may not represent a balance. However, the lab will demonstrate that foods have very different calorie values and careful selection of foods may be required to control the amount of calories ingested. Physical activity also varies with each day, so your recordings will reflect your activity for one day only. A log kept over a longer period of time would be indicative of the balance effect that occurs on a long-term basis.

▶ Laboratory 7

RISKO: Your Chance of Having a Heart Attack

Purpose

To assess your chances of suffering a heart attack based on the interplay of risk factors recognized by the American Heart Association.

Procedure

Follow the directions indicated, then compare your score with the scale that accompanies the game. (Note: The purpose of this game is to yield only an **estimate.**)

RISKO

The game is played by making squares that—from left to right—represent an increase in your RISK FACTORS. These are medical conditions and habits associated with an increased danger of heart attack. Not all risk factors are measurable enough to be included in this game; see back of sheet for other *RISK FACTORS.*

Rules

Study each RISK FACTOR and its row. Find the box applicable to you and circle the large number in it. For example, if you are 37, circle the number in the box labeled 31–40.

After checking out all the rows, add the circled numbers. This total—your score—is an estimate of your risk.

Heredity

Count parents, grandparents, brothers, and sisters who have had heart attack and/or stroke.

AGE	10 to 20	21 to 30	31 to 40	41 to 50	51 to 60	61 to 70 and over
HEREDITY	No known history of heart disease	1 relative with cardiovascular disease Over 60	2 relatives with cardiovascular disease Over 60	1 relative with cardiovascular disease Under 60	2 relatives with cardiovascular disease Under 60	3 relatives with cardiovascular disease Under 60
WEIGHT	More than 5 lbs. below standard weight	−5 to +5 lbs. standard weight	6-20 lbs. over weight	21-35 lbs. over weight	36-50 lbs. over weight	51-65 lbs. over weight
TOBACCO SMOKING	Non-user	Cigar and/or pipe	10 cigarettes or less a day	20 cigarettes a day	30 cigarettes a day	40 cigarettes a day or more
EXERCISE	Intensive occupational and recreational exertion	Moderate occupational and recreational exertion	Sedentary work and intense recreational exertion	Sedentary occupational and moderate recreational exertion	Sedentary work and light recreational exertion	Complete lack of all exercise
CHOLESTEROL OR FAT % IN DIET	Cholesterol below 180 mg.% Diet contains no animal or solid fats	Cholesterol 181-205 mg.% Diet contains 10% animal or solid fats	Cholesterol 206-230 mg.% Diet contains 20% animal or solid fats	Cholesterol 231-255 mg.% Diet contains 30% animal or solid fats	Cholesterol 256-280 mg.% Diet contains 40% animal or solid fats	Cholesterol 281-300 mg.% Diet contains 50% animal or solid fats
BLOOD PRESSURE	100 upper reading	120 upper reading	140 upper reading	160 upper reading	180 upper reading	200 or over upper reading
SEX	Female under 40	Female 40-50	Female over 50	Male	Stocky male	Bald stocky male

RISKO. © Michigan Heart Association.

Tobacco Smoking

If you inhale deeply and smoke a cigarette way down, add one to your classification. Do *not* subtract because you think you do not inhale or smoke only a half inch on a cigarette.

Exercise

Lower your score one point if you exercise regularly and frequently.

188

Cholesterol or Saturated Fat Intake Level

A cholesterol blood level is best. If you can't get one from your doctor, then estimate honestly the percentage of solid fats you eat. These are usually of animal origin—lard, cream, butter, and beef and lamb fat. If you eat much of this, your cholesterol level probably will be high. The U.S. average, 40%, is too high for good health.

Blood Pressure

If you have no recent reading but have passed an insurance or industrial examination chances are you are 140 or less.

Sex

This line takes into account the fact that men have from 6 to 10 times more heart attacks than women of child-bearing age.

Laboratory 7 Results Sheet

Risk score for AGE is _____

Risk score for HEREDITY is _____

Risk score for WEIGHT is _____

Risk score for SMOKING is _____

Risk score for EXERCISE is _____

Risk score for CHOLESTEROL is _____

Risk score for BLOOD PRESSURE is _____

Risk score for SEX is _____

Total Risk score is _____

If You Score

6–11—Risk well below average   25–31—Risk moderate
12–17—Risk below average   32–40—Risk at a dangerous level
18–24—Risk generally average   41–62—Danger urgent. See your doctor
                                                                  now.

Based On Total Score My Risk Is: (circle one)

Well below average   Below average   Generally average
Moderate risk   Dangerous risk   Danger urgent

RISKO. © Michigan Heart Association.

Name _____

Section _____   Date _____

▶ Laboratory 8

Measurement and Evaluation of Blood Pressure

Blood pressure is the amount of force that the blood exerts against the ar-terial walls. It is expressed in millimeters of mercury. There are two phases of blood pressure—one produced during the *contraction phase of the heart, called the* **systolic pressure;** and the *second produced during the relaxation phase of the heart cycle, called the* **diastolic pressure.** Blood pressure may be measured with instruments called a sphygmomanometer (blood pressure cuff) and a stethoscope. Normal limits range from 110–140 systolic and 60–90 diastolic.

Purpose

To determine individual blood pressure at rest.

Part A—Measurement of Resting Blood Pressure

1. Place the cuff around the subject's upper arm so that the lower edge of the cuff is about 1 to 1½ inches above the bend at the elbow. The arm should be at a right angle and in a relaxed, supported position.

2. Place the diaphragm of the stethoscope firmly over the midpoint at the bend of the elbow (antecubital space), directly over the site of the brachial pulse.

3. Be sure the valve control on the pump is completely shut. Inflate the pres-sure to approximately 160 mm, or approximately 30 mm beyond a bra-chial pulse cutoff.

4. Slowly release the pressure by opening the control valve so that pressure decreases at about 2 to 3 mm per second.

5. While decreasing pressure listen for the following sounds:

    a. a "sharp thud" (the first Korotkoff sound), this is accepted as the level of systolic pressure.

    b. the last sound followed by silence marks the diastolic pressure.

Resting Blood Pressure:

$$systolic = \underline{\hspace{3cm}}$$
$$diastolic = \underline{\hspace{3cm}}$$

Questions

1. What are the ranges for normal blood pressure?

    systolic: from _____ to _____

    diastolic: from _____ to _____

2. What happened to blood pressure after exercising? Why?

3. What long-term benefits does exercise have on blood pressure, and Why?

4. What are at least three dangers of hypertension?

▶ Laboratory 9

Heart Rate as a Measure of Cardiovascular Efficiency and Exercise Intensity

To obtain the greatest aerobic benefits from exercise, the effort must not be too high or too low. Generally, it is always better and safer to exercise too easily rather than too hard. The accepted measure of effort is heart rate in beats per minute. For exercise to be productive it must be performed at a pre-determined level. The Karvonen method of determining ideal training heart rate has been endorsed by the American College of Sports Medicine. The proper intensity is actually a range, rather than a single heart rate. This intensity is based on age and resting heart rate. Follow these procedures to determine resting heart rate and proper training intensity.

Purpose

To determine resting heart rate (RHR) and training rate range.

Part A—Resting Heart Rate

Take heart beat while seated by counting either the carotid pulse (either side of larynx) or the radial pulse (thumb side of wrist) for ten (10) seconds and multiply by six to convert to a minute base (BPM).

RHR   TRIAL 1 _____ BPM

TRIAL 2 _____ BPM

TRIAL 3 _____ BPM

SUM OF 3 TRIALS = _____

AVERAGE RHR   = _____ (sum divided by 3)

Scale for Resting Heart Rate Comparison

```
       |            |            |            |        |
----- 50 ----- 55 ----- 60 ----- 65 ----- 70 ----- 75 ----- 80 ----- 85 ----- 95 ---
    Excellent  |  Very good  |    Good     |   Average  |  Poor  |
```

Part B—Determining Training Heart Rate Intensity Using the Karvonen Method

1. ___220___
    − [   ] age
    ───────
    [   ] estimated maximum heart rate (EMHR)
    [   ] Adjusted rate

2. [   ] EMHR
    [   ] RHR (from part A)
    ────────
    [   ] Adjusted rate
    [   ] Adjusted rate

3. a. × .60   (60%)
    ──────
    [   ] work rate
    [   ] work rate

    b. × .90   (90%)
    ──────
    [   ] work rate
    [   ] work rate

4. a. [   ]
    + _____RHR
    [   ] BPM @ 60% level

    b. [   ]
    + _____RHR
    [   ] BPM @ 90%

5. Training rate range from _____ BPM to _____ BPM

Questions

1. What does this training heart rate mean?

2. What is generally regarded as the *minimal* heart rate necessary to create beneficial results in asymptomatic (normal, healthy people)?

    _____ BPM

3. What should you do if you are unable to sustain your heart rate range for the prescribed time period?

▶ Laboratory 10
Evaluation of Aerobic Fitness

The maximal O_2 consumption for any individual is the best criterion of how well various physiological functions can support the metabolic needs of work, exercise, and daily life. The most limiting factor to an individual's general well-being (fitness) is how much O_2 he/she can process; this is referred to as aerobic capacity, maximum O_2 uptake, or maximum O_2 consumption. Ultimately, it depends on the efficiency of the aerobic pathways, that is, cardiorespiratory efficiency.

There are several methods of ascertaining the efficiency of the C-R system. The most exact and precise methods involve rather complicated laboratory procedures, which prove to be most unsuitable for testing a great number of individuals.

Fortunately, field tests of fitness (aerobic fitness) have been developed that require only a stopwatch and place to run. The most valid of these field tests is Cooper's 1.5-mile run (researchers such as Pollack, Wilmore, and Cooper have found these relationship coefficients between Cooper's field test and laboratory uptake tests: .89, .90, .94, and .97).

Purpose

To determine the level of your cardiorespiratory fitness.

Testing Precautions

Since heart rate and blood pressure cannot be monitored continuously during a field test, a certain risk exists if you take such a test without having been properly conditioned by previous exercise. Consider the following precautions:

1. Don't take a fitness test prior to beginning an exercise program if you're over 30 years of age.

2. Be sure to have a medical examination, as outlined in chapter 3 before you take a fitness test. If you are over 30, it is still safer to postpone the test until you have completed the six-week starter program as described in chapter 6.

3. If you comply with the above, yet experience extreme fatigue, shortness of breath, light-headedness, or nausea during the test, stop immediately. Do not try to repeat the test until your fitness level has been gradually improved through regular exercise. (From *New Aerobics* by Dr. K. H. Cooper, p. 29).

Part A—Administration of Test

The 1.5-mile run is a timed event. Each individual will cover the full distance (1-1/2 miles) as fast as possible. (This may be accomplished by running, run-walk, job, etc.) Since this is a maximum VO_2 assessment, a maximum effort is encouraged.

Where a one-quarter mile track is available for use, the distance will be completed after six laps. The time should be kept to the nearest second.

Part B—Evaluation and Classification of Performance

Find your respective performance time under the appropriate bracket. Then find the fitness category at left.

Fitness Classifications for 1.5 Mile Run

Women				
	Under 30	**30-39**	**40-49**	**50+**
Superior	< 9:45	< 10:30	< 11:00	< 12:00
Excellent	9:45-11:15	10:30-12:00	11:00-12:30	12:01-13:30
Good	11:16-13:00	12:01-14:00	12:31-15:00	13:31-16:30
Fair	13:01-15:30	14:01-16:30	15:01-17:30	16:31-18:30
Poor	15:31-17:30	16:31-18:30	17:31-19:30	18:31-20:30
Very Poor	17:31+	18:31+	19:30+	20:31+

Men				
	Under 30	**30-39**	**40-49**	**50+**
Superior	< 8:45	< 9:30	< 10:00	< 10:30
Excellent	8:45-10:15	9:31-11:00	10:01-11:30	10:31-12:00
Good	10:16-12:00	11:01-13:00	11:31-14:00	12:01-14:30
Fair	12:01-14:30	13:01-15:30	14:01-16:30	14:31-17:00
Poor	14:31-16:30	15:31-17:30	16:31-18:30	17:01-19:00
Very Poor	16:31+	17:31+	18:31+	19:01+

► Laboratory 11

Aerobic Fitness as Determined by a 5-Minute Run

The amount of oxygen that can process, that is, supply, deliver, and use is the single best indicator of health-related fitness status. This measure is referred to as aerobic fitness and can be evaluated in various methods.

One approach developed by Dr. Donald Michielli uses the distance covered in a 5-minute run as the evaluative procedure. This is similar to Dr. Cooper's 1.5-mile run in that both require a "best" or maximum effort. It must be remembered that any maximum effort can be dangerous; therefore, make these considerations before attempting this or any similar effort:

1. If you are over 30 years of age do not perform this measure prior to starting an exercise program.

2. Be certain to have medical clearance to attempt this measure as well as any exercise program.

3. Be certain to warm up before, and cool down after the effort.

4. If extreme fatigue, dizziness, shortness of breath, or nausea are experienced, seek medical aid immediately.

Purpose

To evaluate aerobic capacity

Procedure

1. Warm up appropriately to prepare for the effort.

2. Where a one-quarter mile track is available, it will be easier to determine the distance covered by dividing the track into segments of 110 yards.

3. There is a 5-minute limit to this effort, and one should cover as much distance within this time period as possible.

199

4. Record the distance to the nearest yard as accurately as possible and refer to the chart for performance rating.

5. Be certain to cool down after the effort.

Distance Covered in Yards	Classification
<680	Very Poor
681–900	Poor
901–1125	Fair
1126–1350	Good
1351 +	Excellent

▶ Laboratory 12
Walking and Swimming: Measures of Fitness

Part A

The walking test, covering three miles in the fastest time possible *without running,* can be performed on a track or any accurately measured distance. As with running, take the test on the top of page 202 with similar precautions and only after you have been exercising regularly for six weeks, especially if you are over 30 years of age.

Part B

The swimming test on the bottom of page 202 involves a 12-minute effort covering as much distance as possible measured in yards. Any one stroke or combination of strokes may be used. It would probably be most easily performed in a pool of known dimensions with another person recording the time and distance.

3-Mile Walking Test (No Running)
Time (Minutes)

Fitness Category		13–19	20–29	30–39	40–49	50–59	60+
				Age (years)			
I. Very poor	(men)	>45:00*	>46:00	>49:00	>52:00	>55:00	>60:00
	(women)	>47:00	>48:00	>51:00	>54:00	>57:00	>63:00
II. Poor	(men)	41:01–45:00	42:01–46:00	44:31–49:00	47:01–52:00	50:01–55:00	54:01–60:00
	(women)	43:01–47:00	44:01–48:00	46:31–51:00	49:01–54:00	52:01–57:00	57:01–63:00
III. Fair	(men)	37:31–41:00	38:31–42:00	40:01–44:30	42:01–47:00	45:01–50:00	48:01–54:00
	(women)	39:31–43:00	40:31–44:00	42:01–46:30	44:01–49:00	47:01–52:00	51:01–57:00
IV. Good	(men)	33:00–37:30	34:00–38:30	35:00–40:00	36:30–42:00	39:00–45:00	41:00–48:00
	(women)	35:00–39:30	36:00–40:30	37:30–42:00	39:00–44:00	42:00–47:00	45:00–51:00
V. Excellent	(men)	<33:00	<34:00	<35:00	<36:30	<39:00	<41:00
	(women)	<35:00	<36:00	<37:30	<39:00	<42:00	<45:00

* < Means "less than"; > means "more than."

12-Minute Swimming Test
Distance (Yards) Swum in 12 Minutes

Fitness Category		13–19	20–29	30–39	40–49	50–59	60+
				Age (years)			
I. Very Poor	(men)	>500*	>400	>350	>300	>250	>250
	women)	>400	>300	>250	>200	>150	>150
II. Poor	(men)	500–599	400–499	350–449	300–399	250–349	250–299
	(women)	400–499	300–399	250–349	200–299	150–249	150–199
III. Fair	(men)	600–699	500–599	450–549	400–499	350–449	300–399
	(women)	500–599	400–499	350–449	300–399	250–349	200–299
IV. Good	(men)	700–799	600–699	550–649	500–599	450–549	400–499
	(women)	600–699	500–599	450–549	400–499	350–449	300–399
V. Excellent	(men)	>800	>700	>650	>600	>550	>500
	(women)	>700	>600	>550	>500	>450	>400

* < Means "less than"; > means "more than."

Excerpt(s) from THE AEROBICS PROGRAM FOR TOTAL WELL BEING by Kenneth H. Cooper M.D., M.P.H. Copyright © 1982 by Kenneth H. Cooper. Used by permission of Bantam Books, a division of Bantam Doubleday-Dell-Publishing Group, Inc.

▶ Laboratory 13
The Back Fitness Test

One of the common musculoskeletal problems afflicting adult Americans is low back pain. Most backaches are due to weaknesses in the muscles that support the vertebrae. This can lead to spinal nerve and disc problems, which create the chronic low back syndrome.

Purpose

To perform a single assessment of back fitness relative to the potential of future back problems.

Procedure

Perform the specific tests as described and determine the grades in the four categories.

Part A—The Sit-Up

1. Do not allow anyone to hold your feet down.

2. Be sure to perform the sit-up with adequate padding under your back.

TEST	GRADE I Excellent	GRADE II Average	GRADE III Fair	GRADE IV Poor
A. THE SIT-UP	Able to sit up with knees bent and hands on shoulders.	Able to sit up with knees bent and arms folded across chest.	Able to sit up with knees bent and arms held out straight.	Unable to sit up with knees bent.

Result: Grade _____

From the book *Goodbye Backache,* by Dr. David Imrie with Colleen Dimson. Copyright 1983. Used by permission of the publisher, Arco Publishing/A division of Simon & Schuster, New York.

Part B—The Double Leg Raise

	GRADE I Excellent	GRADE II Average	GRADE III Fair	GRADE IV Poor
B. THE DOUBLE LEG RAISE	Able to keep back flat against the floor while raising the legs 6 inches for 10 counts.	Able to raise the legs for several counts but back curves partway through the test.	Able to lift the legs but back curves immediately when the legs are raised.	Unable to lift both legs for 10 counts and/or lifting legs causes pain.

Result: Grade _____

Part C—The Lateral Trunk Lift

	GRADE I Excellent	GRADE II Average	GRADE III Fair	GRADE IV Poor
C. THE LATERAL TRUNK LIFT	Able to raise the shoulders 12 inches off the floor without difficulty, holding for 10 counts.	Able to raise the shoulders 12 inches off the floor but with difficulty. Cannot hold for 10 counts.	Able to raise shoulders slightly off the floor and with difficulty.	Unable to raise shoulders off the floor.

Result: Grade _____

Part D—The Hip Flexors

1. Be sure to measure both sides, right and left.

	GRADE I Excellent	GRADE II Average	GRADE III Fair	GRADE IV Poor
D. THE HIP FLEXORS	Able to hold one leg firmly against the chest with the other leg flat against the floor.	With effort able to hold one knee against the chest while straightening the other leg flat to the floor.	With one knee fixed firmly against the chest the other leg raises off the floor.	Unable to get one leg firmly against the chest without causing pain or discomfort.

Result: Grade _____

Questions

Based on your results, what considerations should be made in the type of exercise needed to create change or to prevent change (i.e., to promote improvement or to prevent further deterioration)?

Name _____

Section _____ Date _____

Dealing with Stress

In today's complex and rapidly advancing technology, the physical effort required for daily living has been decreased significantly. Due to this ever-increasing pace of life, the human organism is being forced to adapt at a phenomenal rate. People are continually exposed to innumerable visual, auditory, and psychological stimuli to which they must make a variety of responses.

The attempt to deal successfully with these changing situations produces wear and tear on the body called stress. Prolonged stress, unless dealt with effectively, can elicit physiological, psychological, and emotional deterioration. However, when individuals learn to recognize stress the overall effect on the body can be diminished.

Researchers have determined that the body reacts to stress situations in a number of different patterns. It has also been shown that certain individuals exhibit different kinds of "stress symptoms." Stress symptoms that most commonly display themselves include the following: increased heart rate (HR), increased blood pressure (BP), increased respiration rate (RR), increased eye blink rate (EBR), pupil dilation, decreases in hand steadiness, and an increase in muscle tension.

Part A—Measuring Stress

Dr. Thomas Holmes has published his "Social Readjustment Scale", which is a means of quantifying the stresses over a period of time. To determine the amount of stress that has occurred in your life during the last 12 months, simply check the appropriate events on the list provided and total your score. This score can be used to *predict* your chances of suffering illness within the next two years. *It merely gives an indication not a guarantee.*

Reprinted with permission from the *Journal of Psychosomatic Research*, Vol. 11, Holmes and Rahe, "Social Readjustment Rating Scale," 1967, Pergamon Press Ltd., Oxford, England.

Event	Value	Your Score	Event	Value	Your Score
Death of Spouse	100	___	Outstanding personal achievement	28	___
Divorce	73	___	Marital separation	65	___
Death of close family member	63	___	Jail term	63	___
Personal injury or illness	53	___	Spouse begins or stops work	26	___
Marriage	50	___	Starting or finishing school	26	___
Fired from work	47	___	Change in living conditions	25	___
Marital reconciliation	45	___	Revision of personal habits	24	___
Retirement	45	___	Trouble with boss	29	___
Change in family member's health	44	___	Change in work hours conditions	20	___
Pregnancy	40	___	Change in residence	20	___
Sex difficulties	39	___	Change in schools	20	___
Addition to family	39	___	Change in recreational habits	19	___
Business readjustment	39	___	Change in church activities	19	___
Change in financial status	38	___	Change in social activities	18	___
Death of close friend	37	___	Mortgage or loan under $10,000	17	___
Change to different line of work	36	___	Change in sleeping habits	16	___
Change in number of marital arguments	35	___	Change in number of family gatherings	15	___
Mortgage or loan over $10,000	31	___	Vacation		___
Foreclosure of mortgage or loan	30	___	Christmas season	12	___
Change in work responsibilities	29	___	Minor violation of the law	11	___
Son or daughter leaving home	29	___			
Trouble with in-laws	29	___			

Total _____

Part B—Evaluating the Effects of Stress

Total Score:		Result
Less than 150	—	37% chance of becoming ill
150–300	—	51% chance of suffering poor health
More than 300	—	80% chance of illness

Part C—Dealing with Stress

One of the greatest problems is the inability to relax—physically, mentally, and emotionally. If one can learn to relax physically, the simultaneous relaxation effects begin to be achieved emotionally and mentally.

This ability to consciously control body function forms the basis of relaxation techniques like yoga, biofeedback, and transcendental meditation (TM) as well as those developed by Jacobson, Rathbone, and Schade dealing with progressive muscle relaxation.

Dr. Herbert Benson of Harvard Medical School has developed a procedure that produces the same physiological changes as TM.

1. Sit comfortably in a quiet place.

2. Close eyes and relax all muscles.

3. Breathe easily and naturally through your nose. Inhale, then as you exhale say in your mind the word "one." Repeat "one" to yourself each time you breathe out.

4. "One" is a mantra, a mental device to anchor your thoughts. Your thoughts may wander to problems, events, or desires. Try to replace these thoughts with the word "one," and your steady breathing rhythm.

"Meditate" for 10 to 20 minutes, twice daily. Given time and practice the technique will work.

Questions

1. Do you believe it is possible to have "psychological stress" without physiological involvement? If so, how?

2. Explain briefly the statement "one person's stress may be another person's pleasure."

▶ Laboratory 15
Evaluation and Selection
of Activities

Purpose

The purpose of this laboratory is twofold:

1. To evaluate specific physical activities with respect to their fitness benefits.

2. To make tentative decisions concerning physical activities that one might include in one's own life-style.

Part A—Evaluation of Physical Fitness and Selection of Activities

The chart on page 210 lists several popular physical activities. Using the example format, evaluate the potential benefit that one might gain by regular participation in each activity. (Use evaluative scale, 5–3–1–0 to indicate high-average-low-none with respect to potential benefit.) Leave Over-All Benefit column blank.

Part B—Selection of Activities According to Benefits

You now have rated the listed activities with respect to their potential benefits. Hopefully, your ratings were as objective as possible and consistent with the facts pertaining to the physiological, social and emotional effects attendant with regular participation in these activities. Before you can select certain activities that might prove beneficial to you personally, you should now rate the *overall benefit* of each activity. This rating is, of necessity, subjective and should reflect your interest and/or desire to participate in the activity on a regularized basis in the future.

Rate each activity for overall benefit using, 5–3–1–0 for high-moderate-low-or-no benefit, respectively.

Activities   Potential Benefit

	C.V. Endurance	Muscular Endurance	Strength	Flexibility	Balance	Power	Speed	Agility	Reaction Time	Kinesthetic Sense	Mental-Emotional
Golf											
Tennis											
Skiing											
Badminton											
Swimming											
Volleyball											
Basketball											
Bowling											
Football											
Running-Jogging											
Self-Defense											
Handball											
Gymnastics											
Ballet											
Yoga											
Softball											
Fencing											
Archery											
Weight Training											
Calisthenics											
Hiking											
Cycling											
Aerobic Dance											

Now that you have arrived at a total score for each activity, list the six highest-rated activities in descending order.

1. _____

2. _____

3. _____

4. _____

5. _____

6. _____

Your instructor will indicate the activities that are offered by the Department of Physical Education. Hopefully, this information might prove helpful for you in planning your physical activity for future years.

Questions

1. What are three goals of fitness you would like to achieve in the next three months?

    a.

    b.

    c.

2. Which exercises would best help you to achieve your goals?

    a.

    b.

    c.

    d.

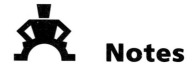 **Notes**

1. H. Kraus, and W. Raab, *Hypokinetic Disease* (Springfield, IL: Charles C Thomas, 1961).

2. *Exercise and Health: A Point of View.* Bureau of Health Education of The American Medical Association.

3. "Exercise," *The New York Times*, Feb. 24, 1981, p. C2.

4. Smoking and Health, Report of the Advisory Committee to the Surgeon General of the Public Health Service, Public Health Service Publication No. 1103, 1964, p. 327.

5. Jane E. Brody, "Latest Data Suggests Exercise Helps Curb Heart Attacks," *New York Times*, March 27, 1979, p. C1.

6. Jane E. Brody, "Study Indicates Moderate Exercise Can Add Years to a Person's Life," *New York Times*, March 6, 1985. p. 1.

7. Ibid., p. 1.

8. A. Kunttiner and T. Somer, "Effects of Muscular Exercise on Plasma Viscosity in Correlation With Post Prandial Triglycerides," *Journal of Applied Physiology*, 18:991–93, 1963.

9. Herbert A. DeVries, *Physiology of Exercise for Physical Education and Athletics* (Dubuque, IA: Wm. C. Brown, 1970), p. 227.

10. R. M. Friedman, M.D. and R. H. Rosenmann, M.D. *Type A Behavior and Your Heart* (New York: Knopf Publishers, 1974), Preface.

11. Karl Menninger, *Love Against Hate* (New York: Harcourt, Brace & World, 1942), p. 169.

12. Dr. Robert Elliott, Is It Worth Dying For? (Bantam Books, 1984).

13. "Women Athletes," *The New York Times Magazine,* May 18, 1980, p. 38.

14. Ibid., p. 38 and 96.

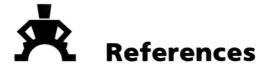

References

"A New Menu to Heal the Heart: A Yearlong Study Proves That Diet, Exercise and Stress Reduction Can Open Arteries and Save Lives." *Newsweek,* July 30, 1990.

"America Shapes Up," *Time,* November 2, 1981.

American College of Sports Medicine: The Recommended Quantity and Quality of Exercise for Developing and Maintaining Fitness in Healthy Adults. Sports Medicine Bulletin, 13:1, 1978.

"Are Americans Fit?, Survey data conflict." *The Physician and Sportsmedicine* 14, no. 11 (November 1986).

Aring, C. D. "On Improving the Public Health." *JAMA* 238 (1978).

Astrand, P.-O., and K. Rodahl. *Textbook of Work Physiology.* 2 ed. New York: McGraw-Hill, 1977.

Avery, C. S. "Abdominal Obesity: Scaling Down This Deadly Risk." *The Physician and Sportsmedicine* 19, no. 10 (October 1991).

Barnard, R. J. "The Heart Needs Warm-up Time." *Physician and Sportsmedicine,* April, 1975.

Blackburn, G., M.D. "Body Composition." *Physician and Sportsmedicine,* March, 1981.

Blair, S. J., H. W. Kohl, et.al. "Physical Fitness and All-Cause Mortality." *JAMA* 262, no. 17 (November 1989).

Bogert, L. J. *Nutrition and Physical Fitness.* Philadelphia: W. B. Saunders Co., 1960.

Bowerman, W. J. and W. E. Harris. *Jogging.* New York: Grosset and Dunlap, 1967.

Casperson, C. J., et. al. *Status of the 1990 Physical Fitness and Exercise Objectives—Evidence from NHIS, 1985.* Public Health Report 101, 1986.

Cooper, K. H., M.D. *Aerobics.* New York: M. Evans & Co., 1968.

Cooper, K. H., M.D. *The New Aerobics.* New York: M. Evans & Co., 1970.

Cooper, K. H., M.D. *The Aerobics Way.* New York: M. Evans & Co., 1978.

Cooper, K. H., M.D. *The Aerobics Program for Total Well-being,* New York: M. Evans & Co., 1982.

Cooper, M. and K. H., M.D. *Aerobics for Women.* New York: M. Evans & Co., 1972.

Corbin, C. et. al. *Concepts in Physical Education.* 2d ed. Dubuque, IA: Wm. C. Brown, 1974.

Costill, D. L., Ph.D., "Quality Training." *The Runner.* May, 1984.

Davis, E. C., et. al. *Biophysical Values of Muscular Activity.* Dubuque, IA: Wm. C. Brown, 1965.

DeMoss, V. "The Fad Diet Guide." *Runners World,* May, 1981.

DeVries, H. *Physiology of Exercise for Physical Education and Athletics.* 2d ed. Dubuque, IA: Wm. C. Brown, 1966.

DiGennaro, J. *Individualized Exercise and Optimal Physical Fitness.* Philadelphia: Lea & Febiger, 1974.

Dominguez, R. H., M.D., *The Complete Book of Sports Medicine.* New York: Scribner's, 1979.

Face the Fats: Understanding the Role of Fats and Cholesterol in Heart Disease. Dept. of Consumer Affairs, Wegmans Food/Pharmacy, Rochester, NY, 1988.

Falls, H. B., et. al. *Foundations of Conditioning.* New York: Academic Press, 1970.

Fiatarone, M. A., et. al. "High Intensity Strength Training in Nonagenarians: Effects on Skeletal Muscle." *JAMA* 263, no. 22 (1990).

Fox, E. L. and D. Mathews. *The Physiological Basis of Physical Education and Athletics.* Philadelphia: W. B. Saunders Co., 1976.

Gilmore, C. P. "Taking Exercise to Heart." *N.Y. Times Magazine,* March 27, 1977.

Goldfine, H., et. al. "Exercising to Health." *The Physician and Sportsmedicine* 19, no. 6 (June 1991).

Grooes, D. "Is Childhood Obesity Related to TV Addiction?" *Physician and Sportsmedicine* 16, no. 11 (November 1988).

Hage, P. "Perceived Exertion: One Measure of Exercise Intensity." *The Physician and Sportsmedicine* 9, no. 9 (September 1981).

Hamilton, E. M. and E. N. Whitney. *Nutrition: Concepts and Controversies.* 2d ed. New York: West Publishing Co., 1982.

Harris, S. S., et. al. "Physical Activity Counseling for Healthy Adults as a Primary Preventive Intervention in the Clinical Setting: Report for the US Preventives Services Task Force." *JAMA* 261, no. 24 (1989).

Hockey, R. V. *Physical Fitness: Pathway to Healthful Living.* St. Louis: C. V. Mosby Co., 1973.

Huse, D. M., M.S., R.D., "Dietary Guidelines for Athletes." *The Physician and Sportsmedicine,* April, 1982.

"In Activity Therapy Patients Literally Move Toward Mental Health." *The Physician and Sportsmedicine,* July, 1977.

Johnson, P. B., et. al. *Physical Education—A Problem Solving Approach to Health and Fitness.* New York: Holt, Rinehart and Winston, 1966.

Karpovich, P. and W. E. Sinning. *Physiology of Muscle Activity.* Philadelphia: W. B. Saunders, Co., 1971.

Katch, F. I. and Wm. D. McArdle. *Nutrition, Weight Control and Exercise.* 3d ed. Philadelphia: Lea and Febiger, 1988.

Kenny, W. L. "Heat Stress Primer." *Fitness Management,* September-October, 1985.

Klafs, C. E. and D. D. Arnkeim. *Modern Principles of Athletic Training.* St. Louis: C. V. Mosby Co., 1963.

"Liquid Diets: Are They Safe, How They Work." *Newsweek,* April 30, 1990.

Marley, Wm. P., M.D. *Health and Physical Fitness.* Philadelphia: Saunders College Publishing Co., 1982.

McArdle, Wm. D., et. al. *Exercise Physiology: Energy, Nutrition and Human Performance.* Philadelphia: Lea & Febiger, 1981.

Miller, D. K. and T. E. Allen, *Fitness: A Lifetime Commitment.* Minnesota: Burgess Publishing, 1986.

Nash, H., "Reemphasizing the Role of Exercise in Preventing Heart Disease." *The Physician and Sportsmedicine* 17, no. 3 (March 1989).

Perry, P., et. al., "Total Fitness, '85." *The Runner,* April, 1985.

"Physical Exercise: An Important Factor for Health." International Federation of Sportsmedicine Position Statement, *The Physician and Sportsmedicine* 18, no. 3 (March 1990).

Piscopo, J. *Fitness and Aging.* New York: J. Wiley & Sons Publishing.

Promoting Health/Preventing Disease: Year 2000 Objectives for the Nation. Department of Health and Human Services, Washington, D.C., 1990.

Reid, J. G. and J. M. Thomson. *Exercise Prescription for Fitness.* New Jersey: Prentice-Hall, 1985.

"Running Away From Worries." *Runners World Magazine,* Oct., 1973.

Sharkey, B. J. *Physiology of Fitness.* Champaign, IL: Human Kinetics, 1979.

Stephens, T., Ph.D. "Health Status Surveys of the National Center for Health Statistics." *Preventive Medicine,* 1988.

Stockton, W. "Can Exercise Alter the Aging Process?" *New York Times,* November 28, 1988.

Stockton, W. "When Exercise Isn't Enough." *New York Times,* February 20, 1989.

"Television Viewing as a Health Hazard to Children." *American Academy of Pediatrics Television Committee,* 1990.

"The Health Benefits of Exercise." *The Physician and Sportsmedicine* 15, no. 10 (October 1987).

The Health Letter. "Exercise While You Diet." Vol. VII, No. 5, March 12, 1976.

Van Huss, W. D., et. al. *Physical Activity in Modern Living.* 2d ed. New Jersey: Prentice-Hall, Inc., 1969.

Vitale, F. *Individualized Fitness Programs.* New Jersey: Prentice-Hall, Inc., 1973.

"Weighing the Facts on Obesity," *Worldview,* vol. 4, no. 1, Nestle Information Service, Washington, D.C.

Wilkinson, J. F., M.D. *Don't Raise Your Child to be a Fat Adult.* New York: Bobbs-Merrill Co., Inc., 1980.

Williams, M. H. *Nutrition for Fitness and Sports.* Dubuque, IA: Wm. C. Brown Company.

Wolf, M. D. *The Complete Book of Nautilus Training.* Chicago: Contemporary Books, Inc., 1984.

Wood, P., D. Sc. "You Can Lose Weight Safely." *Runners World Magazine,* January, 1985.

Work, J. A. "Strength Training: A Bridge to Independence for the Elderly." *The Physician and Sportsmedicine* 17, no. 11 (November 1989).

"Young Women are Getting Fatter, Study Finds." *New York Times,* Science Section, February 23, 1989.

Zohman, L., M.D., *Exercise Your Way to Fitness and Heart Health.* New Jersey: Best Foods, CPC International, 1974.

Index

219